PHYSICAL THERAPIST
Examination Review

VOLUME I

Ninth Edition

PHYSICAL THERAPIST
Examination Review

VOLUME I

Ninth Edition

Theresa Meyer, PT

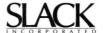

6900 Grove Road Thorofare, NJ 08086

Publisher: John H. Bond
Editorial Director: Amy E. Drummond
Senior Associate Editor: Jennifer L. Stewart

Meyer, Theresa
        Physical therapist examination review / Theresa Meyer.
            v. <1->. cm.
        Includes bibliographical references.
        ISBN 1-55642-474-4 (set : alk. paper).
            1-55642-471-X (Vol. 1)
            1-55642-485-X (Vol. 2)
            1-55642-468-X (Disk)
        1. Physical therapy--Outlines, syllabi, etc. 2. Physical therapy--Examinations, questions, etc. I. Title.

        RM701.6 .M49 2000
        615.8'2'076--dc21   00-027002

Printed in the United States of America.
Published by: SLACK Incorporated
                   6900 Grove Road
                   Thorofare, NJ 08086-9447 USA
                   Telephone: 856-848-1000
                   Fax: 856-853-5991
                   www.slackbooks.com

Last digit is print number: 10 9 8 7 6 5 4 3 2 1

Dedication

In memory of my grandmother, Margaret Anna Liss.

Contents

About the Author

Theresa Meyer, BS, PT received her physical therapy degree from Thomas Jefferson College of Allied Health in 1986. She also received a BA degree in health and physical education from Messiah College in 1984.

Theresa started her career as a traveling physical therapist for Pro Therapy of America. This experience allowed her to gain valuable insight into a wide variety of health care settings, including home health, long-term care, outpatient facilities, as well as acute and rehabilitation hospitals. This also provided exposure to many health care systems throughout the United States.

She attended the World Physical Therapy Conference in Sydney, Australia in 1986 to further her education of physical therapy and research internationally. At this time, she wrote the most widely used physical therapy review books for the board licensure examination. This project was born out of a desire to assist with the stress and time constraints that physical therapy students undergo in preparation for the national board licensure examination. Theresa Meyer's *Review Book for the Physical Therapy Licensing Exam*, was the first book on the market to assist the student in exam preparation. She also wrote the *Review Book for the Physical Therapist Assistant*, which offered a multipurpose approach to assist physical therapist assistant students in studying for the board exam and comprehensive finals. Both books are best-sellers and have been used as textbooks in the United States and internationally. The books evolved through many updates and revisions to become two-volume sets with the addition of a software program to simulate computer examination testing in the current examination format.

In 1987, Theresa Meyer founded, and is the owner of, Midwest Hi-Tech Publishers. In 1988, Pro Therapy promoted her to Director of Rehabilitation at Three Rivers Area Hospital in Michigan. She developed cardiac rehabilitation, sports medicine, and fitness programs for the hospital while managing both inpatient and outpatient programs. She also served as their Regional Director for Southwest Michigan. She intertwined her responsibilities at the hospital with a consultant position to additional hospitals and outpatient facilities in the areas of new program development, clinic management, personnel hiring, staff education and preparation for JCAHO and Medicare reviews.

At this time, Theresa was attending many American Physical Therapy conventions to accelerate her learning in physical therapy. Her next career step was cofounding Physical Therapy and Sports Medicine Centers, a private practice that grew from one clinic in 1990 to 10 clinics. The private practices provided Michigan communities with state-of-the-art facilities and highly trained staff. She wrote a *Guide to Evaluation with Forms for the Physical Therapist* to provide physical therapists a succinct and easy method to perform comprehensive examinations of patients. She also worked as an educator for Pro Exam Source, teaching review workshops for the licensing examination to physical therapists and physical therapist assistants.

She sold her private practices to a national corporation in 1997 and retired. In 1998, she was a cofounder in Outpatient Certification Consultants. She and her partner wrote a new manual for Medicare certification, *Outpatient Policy and Procedure Manual*, to assist clinics in preparing for Medicare certification and meeting health care guidelines. Currently, she resides in Michigan and is working as a consultant and author.

Preparing for the Examination and Instructions for Use of These Review Books

1. Passing exam scores will vary by state. Be sure to check with the state in which you are taking your exam, or plan on working in, for their guidelines on passing scores. Some states will also require a jurisprudence examination on the rules, laws, and regulations governing physical therapy in that state, a test of English language proficiency, AIDS training, credential evaluation, and a supervised practice period. Check with the state you will be practicing in to determine what is necessary for licensure.

2. Study ahead of time systematically utilizing the review books as follows:
   - Study one chapter at a time.
   - Review Volume I and Volume II systematically.
   - Do not skip from mid-chapter to another. You may study chapters in the order that best fits your needs. For example, reviewing areas of strength first and proceeding to areas that require more time.
   - If you have class notes that you feel are pertinent and the information is not included in these books, then integrate them into these chapters.

3. After studying all the chapters, proceed to the sample test questions, first in the books, then on the computer disk. Answer all questions, 1 through 200, in 4 hours.

4. If several questions are missed in one area, further research is recommended utilizing the bibliography list or restudying the review book chapters.

5. Visit the site of the examination prior to the test to become acquainted with its location and parking.

6. Recheck for all documents necessary to take the exam: identification, ID with photo, and signature on identification.

7. Please note this review book is intended to assist in preparing for the state licensure exam. Since many factors (eg, adequate preparation time, educational foundation, study habits, etc) contribute to passing the exam/finals, studying the review books alone does not guarantee passing the examination/finals.

8. Do not cram for the exam the night before but get a good night's rest instead. On the morning of the exam, eat a healthy breakfast and plan to leave so you arrive at the site 15 to 20 minutes early. Think positively and good luck!

Chapter One
Gross Anatomy

Muscle Actions

Shoulder

Flexion
Deltoid—anterior
Biceps
Pectoralis major
Coracobrachialis

Extension
Deltoid—posterior
Triceps—long head
Teres major
Latissimus dorsi

Abduction
Deltoid—middle
Supraspinatus
Biceps—long head

Adduction
Pectoralis major
Teres major
Biceps—short head
Coracobrachialis
Latissimus dorsi
Triceps—long head

Lateral Rotation
Infraspinatus
Teres minor
Deltoid—posterior
Pectoralis major

Medial Rotation
Subscapularis
Teres major
Deltoid—anterior

Elbow

Flexion
Biceps
Brachialis

Extension
Triceps
Anconeus

Brachioradialis
Extensor carpi radialis longus
Pronator teres
Palmar longus
Flexor carpi radialis
Flexor carpi ulnaris

Forearm

Pronation
Brachioradialis
Pronator teres
Pronator quadratus
Flexor carpi radialis

Supination
Biceps
Brachioradialis
Supinator

Wrist

Extension
Extensor carpi radialis longus
Extensor carpi radialis brevis
Extensor carpi ulnaris
Extensor digitorum
Extensor pollicis longus

Flexion
Flexor carpi radialis
Flexor pollicis longus
Flexor carpi ulnaris
Abductor pollicis longus
Palmaris longus
Flexor digitorum superficialis
Flexor digitorum profundus

Abduction
Extensor carpi radialis longus
Extensor carpi radialis brevis
Extensor pollicis brevis
Extensor pollicis longus
Extensor digitorum
Flexor carpi radialis
Abductor pollicis longus

Adduction
Extensor carpi ulnaris
Flexor carpi ulnaris

Scapula

Elevation
Upper trapezius
Serratus anterior—upper
Rhomboids
Levator scapulae

Depression
Lower trapezius
Serratus anterior—lower

Abduction
Serratus anterior

Adduction
Middle trapezius
Rhomboids

Lateral Rotation Upward
Trapezius
Serratus anterior

Medial Rotation Downward
Levator scapulae
Rhomboids

Finger Digits

Thumb extension

Extensor pollicis longus/
brevis

Metacarpalphalangeal (MCP)
abduction
Thumb adduction
Thumb abduction
MCP flexion
Interphalangeal (IP) flexion
Opposition
2nd to 5th digit proximal interphalangeal (PIP) flexion
2nd to 3rd digit distal interphalangeal (DIP) flexion
2nd to 3rd MCP flexion
2nd to 3rd digit MCP with IP
extension

Abduction pollicis longus

Adduction pollicis
Abduction pollicis brevis
Flexor pollicis brevis
Flexion pollicis longus
Opponens pollicis
Flexor digitorum sublimis

Flexor digitorum profundus

Lumbricales
Extensor digitorum commu-
nis
Extensor digiti quintiproprius

Neck

Flexion
Sternocleidomastoid
Longus capitis
Longus colli
Scalenus anterior
Rectus capitis anterior
Platysma

Extension
Upper trapezius
Semispinalis capitis
Splenius capitis
Splenius cervicis
Longissimus capitis
Longissimus cervicis

Lateral Flexion
Longus colli
Rectus capitis lateralis

Obliquus capitis superior
Splenius cervicis

Scalenus anterior
Scalenus medius
Scalenus posterior
Sternocleidomastoid

Splenius capitis
Upper trapezius
Longissimus capitis
Iliocostalis—cervical

Rotation—Same Side
Longus colli
Longus capitis
Rectus capitis anterior
Rectus capitis posterior
Obliquus capitis inferior
Splenius cervicis
Splenius capitis
Longissimus capitis

Rotation—Opposite Side
Sternocleidomastoid
Scalenus anterior
Scalenus posterior
Scalenus medius
Upper trapezius
Semispinalis cervicis
Cervical multifidus
Cervical rotators

Temporomandibular Joint (TMJ)

Protraction
Pterygoideus medialis (internus)

Elevation
Masseter temporalis
(pterygoideus medialis
internus)

Pterygoideus lateralis (externus)

Trunk/Back

Flexion
Rectus abdominis
Internal oblique
External oblique

Extension
Erector spinae
Longissimus throacis
Quadratus lumborum
Iliocostalis lumborum

Rotation
External oblique
Internal oblique
Intercostal (8-12)
Iliohypogastric
Rectus abdominis

Latissimus dorsi
Semispinalis
Multifidus
Rotators

Elevation of the Pelvis
Internal oblique
External oblique
Quadratus lumborum
Ilicostalis lumborum

Hip

Flexion
Psoas major
Iliacus
Sartorius
Rectus femoris
Tensor fasciae latae
Gluteus minimus
Pectineus
Adductor magnus—anterior
Adductor brevis
Adductor longus

Extension
Semimembranosus
Semitendinosus
Biceps femoris—long head
Piriformis
Adductor magnus—posterior
Gluteus medius—posterior
Gluteus maximus

Medial Rotators
Adductor longus
Adductor brevis
Gluteus minimus
Gluteus medius—anterior
Semimembranosus
Semitendinosus
Tensor fasciae latae

Lateral Rotators
Psoas major
Iliacus
Sartorius
Internal obturator
External obturator
Gluteus medius—posterior
Gluteus maximus
Gemellus—superior
Gemellus—inferior
Quadratus femoris
Biceps femoris—long head
Piriformis

Abduction
Tensor fasciae latae
Gluteus minimus
Gluteus medius
Gemelli—inferior

Adduction
Adductor longus
Adductor brevis
Adductor magnus
Pectineus

Gemelli—superior
Obturator—internal
Piriformis
Iliacus
Sartorius
Psoas major

Gracilis
Gluteus maximus—lower
Obturator—external

Knee

Flexion
Semimembranosus
Semitendinosus
Biceps femoris
Sartorius
Gracilis
Popliteus
Plantaris
Gastrocnemius

Extension
Rectus femoris
Vastus lateralis
Vastus intermedius
Vastus medialis

Medial Rotation
Sartorius
Gracilis
Popliteus
Semimembranosus
Semitendinosus

Lateral Rotation
Biceps femoris

Ankle

Inversion
Tibialis—anterior
Tibialis—posterior
Flexor hallucis longus
Flexor digitorum longus
Extensor hallucis longus

Eversion
Peroneus brevis
Peroneus longus
Peroneus tertius
Extensor digitorum longus

Dorsiflexion
Tibialis anterior
Peroneus tertius
Extensor digitorum longus
Extensor hallucis longus

Plantar Flexion
Tibialis posterior
Peroneus brevis
Peroneus longus
Plantaris

Soleus
Gastrocnemius
Flexor digitorum longus
Flexor hallucis longus

Toes

Great toe MIP extension	Extensor hallucis longus
Great toe IP flexion	Flexor hallucis longus
Great toe MIP flexion	Flexor hallucis brevis
2nd to 5th digit MIP extension	Extensor digitorum longus
2nd to 5th digit DIP flexion	Flexor digitorum longus
2nd to 5th digit PIP flexion	Flexor digitorum brevis
Toe abduction PIP	Dorsal interossei
Toe adduction PIP	Plantar interossei

Muscles of the Head, Face, and Scalp Region

Muscle	Function
Auricularis—anterior	Draws the ear forward and downward
Auricularis—posterior	Elevates and retracts the ear
Auricularis—superior	Slightly elevates the ear
Buccinator	Aids in chewing food and compressing the cheeks
Corrugator	Causes the eyebrows to draw medially and downward (eg, causes a frowning expression)
Depressor anguli oris	Depresses the angle of the mouth (eg, causes a grieving expression)
Depressor labii inferior	Depresses the lower lip
Depressor septi	Causes the nostrils to close inward
Pterygoideus lateralis	Assists in chewing and protrusion
Levator anguli oris	Elevates the corners of the mouth
Levator labii superiores	Elevates the upper lip
Nasalis	Enlarges or compresses the nostrils, causing them to either flare in or flare out
Masseter	Clenches the teeth, elevates the jaw, assists in chewing

Pterygoideus medialis	Elevates and protracts the lower jaw, assists in chewing
Mentalis	Causes the lower lip to protrude and rise (eg, causes an expression of doubtfulness)
Orbicularis oris	Causes the lips to protrude and compress
Occipitofrontalis	Moves the scalp backward and forward (eg, raises eyebrows, causes a surprised expression)
Orbicularis oculi	Assists in closing the eyelids
Procerus	Causes the eyebrows to draw down and in medially
Risorius	Causes the mouth to retract backward (eg, causes a grinning face)
Temporalis	Elevates the jaw and clenches the teeth
Temporoparietalis	Draws back the skin of the temples (eg, tightens the scalp)
Zygomaticus	Causes the mouth's angles to draw upward and backward (eg, causes a laughing face)

Chart of Combined Actions to be Tested With Muscles

Action	Muscle
Shoulder shrug, scapular upward rotation	Upper trapezius
Shoulder protraction and scapular upward rotation	Serratus anterior
Scapular elevation and downward rotation	Levator scapula
Scapular adduction, elevation, downward rotation	Rhomboids
Shoulder abduction with lateral rotation	Supraspinatus, infraspinatus
Shoulder adduction with medial rotation	Latissimus dorsi, teres major, and subscapular
Shoulder abduction, flexion, extension	Deltoid
Hip flexion, abduction, lateral rotation	Sartorius
Hip flexion, abduction, medial rotation	Tensor fascia lata
Hip extension, knee flexion, and leg lateral rotation	Biceps femoris
Hip extension, knee flexion, and leg medial rotation	Semitendinosus Semimembranous

Innervation of Muscles

Upper Exremity

Muscle	Nerve	Origin
Biceps	Musculocutaneous	C5, C6
Brachialis	Musculocutaneous	C5, C6
Coracobrachialis	Musculocutaneous	C6, C7
Deltoid	Axillary	C5, C6
Infraspinatus	Suprascapular	C4, C5, C6
Latissimus dorsi	Thoracodorsal	C6, C7, C8
Levator scapulae	Cervical 3 and 4, dorsal scapular	C4, C5
Pectoralis major	Lateral and medial pectoral	C5, C6, C7
Pectoralis minor	Medial pectoral	C7, C8, T1
Rhomboid major	Dorsal scapular	C4, C5
Rhomboid minor	Dorsal scapular	C4, C5
Serratus anterior	Long thoracic	C5,C6,C7,C8
Sternocleidomastoid	Cranial nerve XI	C1,C2,C3,C4
Subclavius	Subclavian	C5, C6
Subscapularis	Upper/lower subscapular	C5, C6, C7
Supraspinatus	Suprascapular	C4, C5, C6
Teres major	Lower subscapular	C5, C6, C7
Teres minor	Axillary	C5, C6
Trapezius	Cranial nerve XI, ventral ramus	C2, C3, C4

Chart of the Three Primary Hand/Forearm Nerves

Radial Nerve (C5, C6, C7, C8)	Medial Nerve (C6, C7, C8, T1)	Ulnar Nerve (C7, C8, T1)
Abductor pollicis longus	Flexor pollicis longus	Opponens digiti minimi
Anconeus	Palmaris longus	Palmar brevis
Brachialis	Lumbricales1 & 2	Lumbricales 3 & 4
Brachioradialis	Flexor digitorum superficialis	Flexor carpi ulnaris
Extensor carpi Radialis longus	Pronator quadratus	Flexor digiti minimi
Extensor carpi ulnaris		
Extensor digitorum longus		Abductor digiti minimi
Extensor digitorum minimi		
Extensor indicis proprius	Opponens pollicis	
Extensor pollicis brevis	Abductor pollicis brevis	
Extensor pollicis longus	Flexor carpi radialis	Adductor pollicis
Supinator	Pronator teres	Interossei
Triceps	Flexor digitorum profundus 2 & 3	Flexor digitorum profundus 4 & 5

Radial nerve: the largest branch of the brachial plexus, arising on each side as a continuation of the posterior cord.

Medial nerve: a branch of the brachial plexus that, along with the lateral pectoral nerve, supplies the pectoral muscles.

Ulnar nerve: one of the terminal branches of the brachial plexus that arises on each side from the medial cord of the plexus.

Trunk

Muscle group	Innervation Level
Rectus abdominis	T7 to 12
Internal oblique	T7 to L1
External oblique	T5 to 11

Lower Extremity

Muscle Group	Innervation Level
Sartorius	L1 to 3
Adductors	L2 to 4
External rotators	L3 to S2
Tensor fasciae latae	L4 to S1
Hamstrings	L4 to S3
Quadriceps	L2 to 4
Anterior tibialis	L4 to 5
Gastrocnemius	L5 to S1
Flexor hallucis longus	S1 to 2
Extensor digitorum brevis	S2 to 3

Lower Extremity Innervation

Tibial Nerve (L4, L5, S1, S2, S3)

Plantaris
Gastrocnemius
Popliteus
Soleus
Posterior tibialis
Flexor digitorum longus
Flexor hallucis longus

The Tibial Nerve Divides Into:

Lateral Plantar Nerve	**Medial Plantar Nerve**
Dorsal interossei	Flexor digitorum brevis
Plantar interossei	Flexor hallucis brevis
Abductor digiti minimi	Abductor hallucis
Flexor digiti minimi	Lumbricales 1
Opponens digiti minimi	

Quadratus plantae
Lumbricales 2, 3, and 4
Adductor hallucis

The Common Peroneal Nerve (L4, L5, S1, S2)

Superficial Peroneal Nerve
Peroneus longus
Peroneus brevis

Deep Peroneal Nerve
Tibialis anterior
Peroneus tertius
Extensor hallucis longus
Extensor digitorum longus
Extensor digitorum brevis

Femoral Nerve (L2, L3, L4)

Iliacus
Pectineus
Sartorius
Rectus femoris
Vastus medialis
Vastus lateralis
Vastus intermedius

Sciatic Nerve (L4, L5, S1, S2, S3)
Biceps femoris
Semitendinosus
Semimembranosus
Adductor magnus

Superior Gluteal (L4, L5, S1)
Gluteus medius
Gluteus minimus
Tensor fasciae latae

Inferior Gluteal (L5, S1, S2)
Gluteus maximus

Obturator Nerve (L2, L3, L4)
Obturator—external
Adductor brevis
Adductor longus
Adductor magnus
Gracilis

Lumbar Plexus (L1, L2, L3, L4)
Psoas major
Psoas minor

Sacral Plexus (L4, L5, S1, S2, S3)
Piriformis
Obturator—internal
Quadratus femoris
Gemelli—superior and inferior

Muscles with Dual Innervation

Muscle	Nerves
Flexor digitorum profundus	Median nerve—digits 1 and 2 Ulnar nerve—digits 3 and 4
Flexor pollicis brevis	Median nerve Ulnar nerve—deep head of muscle
Adductor magnus	Sciatic nerve Obturator nerve
Lumbricales—hand	Median nerve—digits 1 and 2 Ulnar nerve—digits 3 and 4

Common Muscle Attachments

Upper Extremity

Greater Tuberosity of Humerus
Supraspinatus
Infraspinatus
Teres minor

Lesser Tuberosity of Humerus
Subscapularis

Medial Epicondyle of Humerus
Common flexor tendon's origin
Common injury is golf elbow

Lateral Epicondyle of Humerus
Common extensor tendon's origin
Common injury is tennis elbow

Lower Extremity

ASIS—Anterior Superior Iliac Spine
Sartorius

Anterior Inferior Iliac Spine
Rectus femoris

Greater Trochanter
Gluteus minimus
Gluteus medius
Piriformis
Obturator—internal
Gemelli—inferior and superior

Lesser Trochanter
Psoas major

Ischial Tuberosity
Semitendinosus
Semimembranosus
Biceps femoris
Adductor magnus

Iliac Crest
Tensor fasciae latae

Pubic Ramus
Pectineus
Adductor magnus
Gracilis
Adductor brevis

Medial Femoral Condyle
Gastrocnemius

Lateral Femoral Condyle
Popliteus

Navicular Tubercle
Tibialis posterior

Joint Integrity

Shoulder Joint

Ball and socket joint/enarthrodial joint
1. Coracoclavicular ligament: connects the clavicle and coracoid process of the scapula.
   a.   Trapezoid ligament
   b.   Conoid ligament
2. Acromioclavicular ligament: located at the outer end of the clavicle and connects to the acromion process of the scapula.
   a.   Inferior ligament
   b.   Superior ligament
3. Coracohumeral ligament: from the coracoid process, it connects to the greater tuberosity of the humerus.

Elbow Joint

Hinge joint/ginglymus joint
1. Orbicular ligament: surrounds the head of the radius.
2. Radial collateral: restricts lateral displacement of the elbow joint.
3. Ulnar collateral: restricts medial displacement of the elbow joint.

Hip Joint

Ball and socket joint/enarthrodial joint
1. Iliofemoral ligament: y-shaped ligament that limits extension of the hip.
2. Pubofemoral ligament: limits extension of the hip.
3. Ischiofemoral ligament: limits anterior displacement of the hip.

Knee Joint

Hinge joint/ginglymus joint
1. Anterior cruciate: prevents anterior displacement of the tibia on the femur.
2. Posterior cruciate: prevents posterior displacement of the tibia on the femur.

3. Medial collateral ligament: stabilizes the medial aspect of the knee joint (tibiofemoral joint).
4. Lateral collateral ligament: stabilizes the lateral aspect of the knee joint.
5. Popliteal: provides lateral and posterior support to the knee joint.

Ankle Joint

Hinge joint/ginglymus
1. Deltoid ligament: lateral stability between medial malleolus, navicular bone, talus, and calcaneus.
2. Lateral ligaments: lateral ligament support; injury results in inversion sprain.
   a. Anterior talofibular: secures fibula to talus.
   b. Calcaneofibular: secures fibula to calcaneus.
   c. Posterior talofibular: secures fibula to talus.

Foot

1. Plantar calcaneonavicular ligament (spring ligament): supports the medial aspect of the longitudinal arch.
2. Long plantar ligament: supports the lateral aspect of the longitudinal arch.

Bony Landmarks With Their Corresponding Vertebral Level

Bony Landmark	Vertebral Level
Sacroiliac joint/ posterior superior iliac spine	S2
Sacral promontory	L5, S1
Crest of ilium	L4, L5
Spinal cord ends	L2
Navel, umbilicus	T10
Inferior angle of scapula	7th rib level, T7
Superior angle of scapula	2nd rib level, T7
Bifurcations of the tracheas	T4
Spine of scapula	T3

Chapter Two
Physiology

Fuels For Exercise

1. Three primary food sources are carbohydrates, proteins, and fats. Each food source converts adenosine triphosphate (ATP) energy to exercise.
2. Carbohydrates are the major fuel, utilized first during prolonged, low-intensity and short, high-intensity exercises. Glucose is the end product of CH_2O digestion. Glucose that is not readily needed for energy is stored in muscle cells in the form of glycogen.
3. The basic form of fat used for fuel is called free fatty acid. This is stored in adipose tissue as a triglyceride. This fuel source is utilized after carbohydrates during prolonged, moderate exercises.
4. Proteins are very rarely utilized as a fuel source for exercise.
5. Definition of calorie: the amount of heat it takes to raise the temperature of one kilogram of water 1°C.
6. The amount of calories required in the conversion process to energy is different for protein, carbohydrates, and fats. One gram of CH_2O yields 4 calories. One gram of fat yields 9 calories. One gram of protein yields 4 calories.

Energy Systems

Aerobic System	Versus	Anaerobic System
Oxygen system		Lactic acid
Slow process		Rapid process
Fuel source = fats		Fuel source = Glycogen
Unlimited ATP production		Limited ATP
Low fatigue		Easily fatigued
Long duration activities, long distance		1- to 3-minute activities
		Sprint or high power, short duration
		Byproduct causes fatigue (lactic acid)

Muscle Fibers

Slow Twitch	Versus	Fast Twitch Muscle
High aerobic capacity		Low aerobic capacity
Low anaerobic capacity		High anaerobic capacity
High capillary density		Low capillary density
Slow contraction		Fast contraction
Slow fatigue		Fast fatigue
Long-distance activity		Short-distance activity
Example: Marathon		*Example: Sprinting*

Muscle Contraction

Concentric Contraction

1. Isotonic or dynamic are other names for this contraction.
2. The muscle shortens as it develops tension.

Eccentric Contraction

1. The muscle lengthens as it develops tension.
2. Example: lowering a weight during a hard press is considered a negative repetition or eccentric contraction.

Isotonic

Speed is variable; the muscle will shorten and develop tension.

Isometric

No change in muscle length, but muscle will develop tension.

Isokinetic

Speed is constant; muscle will shorten in length and maintain maximum tension throughout range of motion.

Theory of Specificity of Training

- Specific training patterns will cause specific physiological responses.
- The effects of training are specific to the sport/activity.
- Specific physiological training applies to each sport because each needs different capacities.

Oxygen Transport System

The oxygen transport system is important during endurance exercise. For a successful performance, one must be able to efficiently transport oxygen to the working muscles.

Definition of Terms

- VO_2 = oxygen transported
- SV = stroke volume—amount of blood the heart pumps per beat
- HR = heart rate—beats per minute

Formulas

1. A-VO_2 Diff Arterial Mixed Venous O_2 Difference = oxygen—the muscle extracts from arterial blood; the more extracted, the less venous blood.
2. MAX V0 = SV x HR x AVO_2 Diff

Muscle Soreness Theory

(The following are only theories as to why muscle soreness may occur)

1. Tearing of muscle fibers, which results in tissue damage.
2. Muscle spasms, which reduce blood flow to muscle.
3. Retention of water/inflammation in tissue.
4. Overstretching of connective tissue (epimysium), which surrounds muscle.

Strength Duration Curve

Strength duration curve is a graphic showing the relationship between the intensity (Y axis) and various durations (X-axis) of the threshold electric stimulus for a muscle, with the stimulating cathode positioned over the motor point. The strength duration curve may be utilized to determine if a muscle is innervated, partially innervated, or denervated.

Definitions

Action Potential

A brief regenerative electrical potential that propagates along a single axon or muscle fiber membrane. The action potential is an all-or-none response to a stimulus. When the stimulus is at or above the threshold, the action potential generated has a constant size and configuration.

Chronaxie

The time required for an electrical current twice the rheobase to elicit the first visible muscle twitch.

Epimysium

The connective tissue that surrounds the entire muscle. It provides muscular strength and integrity to the muscle.

Excitability

The capacity to be activated by or react to a stimulus.

Golgi Tendon Organ

Located in the tendons and responds to stretch. The golgi tendon organ complements the muscle spindle, and acts as a safeguard against injury. The golgi tendon tells the muscle to relax if the contraction is too strong and would cause injury.

Latency

Interval between the onset of the stimulus and the response. Peak latency is the interval between the onset of the stimulus and a specified peak of the evoked potential.

Motor Point

The point over a muscle when a muscle contraction may be elicited by a minimal-intensity, short-duration electrical stimulus.

Motor Unit

The motor unit consists of the anterior horn cells, its axon, neuro-muscular junctions, and all of the muscle fibers innervated by the axon. A motor unit or fibers can manifest a fast and slow twitch. It is described as the functional unit of skeletal muscle.

Motor Unit Action Potential

Action potential showing the electrical activity of a single motor unit.

Muscle Spindle

Located in the muscle fibers, a sensory nerve is located in the center portion of the spindle. When a spindle is stretched, the following will occur: the nerve impulse will begin, the rate of the stretch is given, and the magnitude of the stretch is given.

Muscle Stretch Reflex

Activation of a muscle following a stretch of the muscle.

Myofibril

Component of a muscle cell composed of contractible filaments. Contains two basic proteins that give the striated pattern:
1. Actin—thin filaments, attached to the Z line

2. Myosin—thin filaments, called the I band.

Sarcomere: smallest functional unit of myofibril. It is the distance between two Z lines.

Rheobase

The intensity of an electrical current necessary to produce a minimal visible twitch of a muscle when applied to the motor parts.

Resting Membrane Potential

The voltage across the membrane of an excitable cell at rest.

Sliding Filament Theory

A theory of muscular contraction that states when a muscle performs an isotonic contraction action, filaments will slide over myosin filaments toward the sarcomere, creating cross-bridges, overlapping thick and thin filaments with great force.

Smooth Muscle Tissue

Found in vessel and artery walls, various tissues of the vascular system, lungs, and intestinal and reproductive systems. Differs from skeletal muscle, secondary to lack of a cross-striated pattern. It is under involuntary control.

Stimulus

An external stimulus (eg, electrical stimulation) that influences the activity of a cell, tissue, or organism. A threshold stimulus is a stimulus that produces a detectable response.

Striated Muscle

Called striated muscle secondary to arrangement of contractible proteins in the muscle that gives a cross-striation pattern. Under voluntary control and innervated by the somatic nervous system.

Chapter Three
Neuroanatomy & Physiology

Cranial Nerves

Nerve #	Name	Action
1	Olfactory	Smells
2	Optic	Sees
3	Oculomotor	Moves the eyes
4	Trochlear	Moves the eyes and controls the contralateral superior oblique
5	Trigeminal	Chews/sensory to face
6	Abducens	Accommodates, moves eyes
7	Facial	Moves the face—taste/salivates/cries
8	Vestibulocochlear	Hears/regulates balance
9	Glossopharyngeal	Tastes/swallows, monitors carotid, body, and sinuses
10	Vagus	Tastes/swallows
11	Accessory	Turns the head, and lifts the shoulders
12	Hypoglossal	Moves the tongue

Sensory nerves = 1, 2, 8
Motor nerves = 3, 4, 6, 11, 12
Mixed nerves/motor and sensory = 5, 7, 9, 10

Dermatome Distribution

Sensory distribution of the cutaneous nerves

Upper Extremity

C1	Top of head
C2	Temple, forehead, occiput
C3	Neck, posterior cheek
C4	Superior part of chest above axilla (clavicle area)
C5	Lateral aspect of the arm, deltoid muscle region
C6	Anterior arm, lateral side of hand to thumb and index finger
C7	Lateral arm and forearm to index, long, and ring fingers
C8	Middle arm and forearm to long, ring, and little fingers

Trunk

T1	Medial side of forearm to base of little finger
T2	Axillary region
T4	Nipple level
T6	Xiphoid process level
T10	Umbilicus level
T12	Anterior superior iliac crest level

Lower Extremity

L1	Lower abdomen and groin region
L2	Anterolateral thigh (back and front of thigh to knee)
L3	Anteromedial thigh, leg, upper buttock
L4	Medial buttock, lateral thigh, medial leg, dorsum of foot, large toe
L5	Posterior lateral thigh, lateral leg, dorsum of foot, medial half of sole, first to third toes
S1	Lateral plantar surface of foot, posterior thigh and leg
S2	Posterior thigh and leg
S3	Groin, medial thigh to knee
S4-5	Perineum, genitals, lower sacrum

Spinal Segment With Movements to Test

Spinal Segment	Movements to Test
Upper Extremity	
C4	Shoulder shrug
C5	Shoulder abduction, external rotation
C6	Wrist extension, elbow flexion
C7	Wrist flexion, elbow extension
C8	Wrist ulnar deviation
Trunk	
T1	Abduction/adduction of fingers
Lower Extremity	
L2	Hip flexion
L3	Hip flexion, knee extension,
L4	Knee extension, ankle dorsiflexion
L5	Ankle dorsiflexion
S1	Ankle plantar flexion and eversion
S2	Knee flexion, ankle plantar flexion

Levels of Cognitive Functioning
(Rancho Los Amigos Scale)

Level

1   No response: patient is unresponsive to any stimuli and appears to be in a deep sleep.

2   Generalized response: patient occasionally reacts to stimuli but not in a purposeful pattern. Responses are limited and inconsistent.

3   Localized response: patient reacts to stimuli but continues to be inconsistent. May follow simple commands in a delayed manner.

4   Confused/agitated: patient responds to stimuli but he or she is unable to process information purposefully. Patient is in a heightened state of activity and behavior is bizarre.

5   Confused/inappropriate/nonagitated: patient is alert and able to follow very simple commands. However, consistency fluctuates.

6   Confused/appropriate: patient can follow directions but only with direct assistance from another individual.

7   Automatic appropriate: patient goes through daily routine automatically but robot-like with shallow recall of activities.

8   Purposeful/appropriate: patient shows carryover for new learning and needs no supervision once activities are learned. Patient is able to recall and is aware of and responsive to environment.

Central Nervous System (CNS)

Consists of the brain and spinal cord, both of which are protected by bone. The brain lies within the cranial vault and the spinal cord is protected by the vertebral canal. The brain joins the spinal canal at the foramen magnum.

Covering of the Central Nervous System

Underneath the bony covering is an inner covering of membranes called meninges. The meninges consist of three layers:

1. Dura mater
   - Thick, fibrous connective tissue
   - Outermost meningeal layer
   - Surrounds the meningeal arteries and veins
   - Adheres to the skull

2. Arachnoid
   - Fine, filamentous network
   - Middle meningeal layer
   - Bridge between the dura and inner meningeal layer
   - Cerebrospinal fluid circulated in the space
   - Considered the hydraulic cushion for the CNS

3. Pia mater
   - Single thickness
   - Innermost meningeal layer
   - Adheres to the surface of the CNS

Ventricles

There are four ventricles or cavities that are filled with cerebrospinal fluid. Cerebrospinal fluid provides a support system to cushion the brain. It also aids in the exchange of nutrients and waste.

1. Lateral ventricles (2): large irregular-shaped ventricles with anterior, posterior, and inferior horns. They communicate with the third ventricle through the foramen of Monro.

2. Third ventricle: located posterior and deep between the two thalami and communicates with the fourth ventricle through the cerebral aqueduct.

3. Fourth ventricle: located in front of the cerebellum and behind the pons and upper part of the medulla oblongata. They are pyramid shaped. The openings (foramina) of Luschka and Magendie create communication between the fourth ventricle and subarachnoid space.

Divided into Six Parts

1. **Cerebrum:** the cerebrum is also called the telencephalon. The telencephalon and diencephalon together constitute the prosencephalon or forebrain. It consists of grayish matter composed of crests (*gyri*) and fissures (*sulci*). The islands of gray matter within each cerebral hemisphere are called basal ganglia. These form an associated motor system in the subthalamus and midbrain. The central sulcus separates the frontal lobe from the parietal lobe. The lateral central fissure, also called the **fissure of Sylvius**, separates the temporal, frontal, and parietal lobes of the brain. The longitudinal cerebral fissure separates the two hemispheres. The parietal hemisphere consists of six lobes on each side:
   1. The frontal lobe, which controls the motor aspects of speech, emotions, judgments, and primary motor cortex for voluntary muscle activation.
   2. The parietal lobe, which controls integration of sensations, touch, pain, temperature, and prioception.
   3. The temporal lobe, which controls auditory stimuli and language comprehension.

4. The occipital lobe, which controls the visual stimuli.
5. The insula, which assist with visceral function.
6. The limbic system, which controls feeding, aggression, sexual response, and emotions.

2. **Diencephalon:** consists of the thalamus, subthalamus, hypothalamus, and epithalamus. The thalamus contains sensory nuclei and motor nuclei. The subthalamus is involved in the control of pathways for motor, sensory, and reticular functions. The hypothalamus controls and integrates the peripheral autonomic nervous system, endocrine processes, and many somatic functions, such as body temperature, sleep, and appetite. The epithalamus secrets hormones that control the pituitary gland.

3. **Midbrain:** the midbrain is also called the mesencephalon. It is one of the three parts of the brainstem lying just below the cerebrum and just above the pons. It connects the pons to the cerebrum and the midbrain to the cerebellum. It assists with motor control, muscle tone, suppression of pain, vision, hearing, and certain auditory and visual reflexes.

4. **Pons:** connects the medulla oblongata to the midbrain, allowing the ascending and descending tracts to pass information. The pons consists of white matter and a few nuclei and is divided into a ventral and dorsal portion. It assists in modulation of pain and controlling arousal.

5. **Medulla oblongata:** the most vital part of the brain, continuing as the bulbous portion of the spinal cord just above the foramen magnum and separated from the pons by a horizontal groove. It assists in control of head movements, vestibulo-ocular reflexes, voluntary motor control, center for vital functions, such as cardiac, respiratory, and vasomotor.

6. **Cerebellum:** linked to the brain stem by three pairs of peduncles—superior, middle, and inferior. It is located behind the dorsal pons and medulla in the posterior fossa. It assists in controlling equilibrium and regulation of muscle tone, posture, and coordination of voluntary muscular activity.

- The cerebellum, pons, and medulla all lie in the posterior fossa and together are known as the hindbrain or rhombencephalon.

Peripheral Nervous System (PNS)

The PNS consists of nerves referred to as lower motor neurons and ganglia outside the vertebral canal. Forty-three pairs of nerves originate from the CNS and make up the peripheral nervous system. Twelve pairs are cranial nerves, which originate from the brain. Thirty-one pairs are spinal nerves, which originate from the spinal cord. The spinal nerves are divided into the following groups: eight cervical, twelve thoracic, five sacral, five lumbar, and one coccygeal. These spinal nerves correspond to a particular vertebral segment and consist of a ventral and dorsal root, except for C1, which has no dorsal root. The ventral root is an efferent fiber to voluntary muscle, viscera, smooth muscle, and glands. The dorsal root is an afferent fiber that provides sensory receptors from skin, joints, and muscles.

Arteries

1. **Internal carotid:** arteries that arise off of the common carotids and branch to form anterior middle cerebral arteries. Each of two arteries start at the bifurcation of the common carotid arteries, through which blood circulates to many structures and organs in the head.

2. **Vertebral arteries:** arteries branching from the subclavian arteries, arising deep in the neck from the cranial and dorsal subclavian surfaces. They supply the brainstem, cerebellum, occipital lobe, and thalamus.

3. **Circle of Willis:** formed by the interconnection of the internal carotid, anterior cerebral, posterior cerebral, anterior communicating, and posterior communicating arteries.

Covering of Peripheral Nervous System

1. Endoneurium
   - Fine, single layer
   - Covers nerve processes

2. Perineurium
   • Thick membrane
   • Encloses large groups of processes

3. Epineurium
   • Thick, tough layer
   • Surrounds the PNS

PNS has Two Subdivisions

1. Afferent fibers carry sensory impulses to the CNS.

2. Efferent fibers carry motor impulses away from the CNS by cranial or spinal nerves. The efferent division is further divided into two subdivisions based on the type of effector supplied.
   • Somatic nervous system innervates skeletal muscle and is usually under voluntary control.
   • Autonomic nervous system innervates cardiac muscle, smooth muscle, and glands.

Major Ascending Tracts of the Spinal Cord

1. Dorsal Columns
Fasciculus gracilis
Origin: C1 to T6
Function: Discrete somatotropic transfer of touch, vibration, and kinesthesia.

Fasciculus cuneatus
Origin: T5 to C1
Function: Discrete somatotropic transfer of touch, vibration, and kinesthesia.

2. Spinothalamic Tracts
Anterior (ventral)
Origin: Laminae I, IV, V
Function: Somatotropic transfer of affective light touch, pain, and temperature.

Lateral
Origin: Laminae, I, IV, V
Function: Somatotropic transfer of affective light touch, pain, and
            temperature.

3. Spinocerebellar Tracts
Ventral (anterior)
Origin: Dorsal horn
Function: Somatotropic transfer of proprioception.

Dorsal
Origin: L3 to C8
Function: Somatotropic transfer of spinal interneuron activity.

Cuneocerebellar
Origin: C7 to C2
Function: Somatotropic transfer of spinal interneuron activity.

4. Spinobrainstem Tracts
Spinoreticular
Origin: Dorsal horn
Function: Nondiscriminative transfer of touch, proprioception.

Spinotectal
Origin: Dorsal horn
Function: Nondiscriminative transfer of touch, proprioception.

Spino-olivary
Origin: Dorsal horn
Function: Somatotropic transfer of spinal interneuron activity.

Major Descending Tracts of the Spinal Cord

1. Corticospinal Tracts
Lateral corticospinal
Origin: Primary motor and sensory cortex
Function: Controls alpha and gamma motor neurons, modulates 1°
            afferent.

Anterior corticospinal
Origin: Primary and secondary motor cortex, sensory cortex
Function: Controls alpha and gamma motor neurons, modulates 1°
            afferent.

2. Rubrospinal Tract
Origin: Red nucleus
Function: Controls alpha and gamma motor neurons, modulates 1°
            afferent.

3. Tectospinal Tract
Origin: Superior colliculus
Function: Controls alpha and gamma motor neurons.

4. Vestibulospinal Tracts
Lateral vestibulospinal
Origin: Deiters' nucleus
Function: Controls alpha and gamma motor neurons.

Medial longitudinal fasciculus (MLF)
Origin: Vestibulare nuclei
Function: Controls alpha and gamma motor neurons.

5. Reticulospinal Tracts
Somatomotor
Origin: Reticular formation
Function: Controls alpha and gamma motor neurons.

Autonomic
Origin: Reticular formation
Function: Controls autonomic preganglionic neurons.

Sensory
Origin: Raphe nuclei; reticular formation
Function: Modulates 1° afferent.

Autonomic Effects

Parasympathetic

Craniosacral division. Primarily involves the protection, conservation, and restoration of body resources; slows heart rate, increases intestinal peristalsis and gland activity, and relaxes sphincters.

Sympathetic

Thoracolumbar division. Prepares the body for fight or flight responses; accelerates heart rate, constricts blood vessels, and raises blood pressure.

	Parasympathetic	Sympathetic
Bronchi	Constriction	Dilation
Heart	Decreased heart rate	Increased heart rate
Intestines	Increased peristalsis	Decreased peristalsis
Pupil	Constriction	Dilation
Blood pressure	Decreased blood pressure	Increased blood pressure

Motor Pathways

Corticospinal Tract

1. Also called pyramidal tract

2. Responsible for:
   - Voluntary movement
   - Grading motor response for fine movements
   - Inhibiting muscle tone

3. Pathway is originated in motor cortex of brain, travels down the corticospinal tract to the brain stem, crosses over in the medulla, pyramidaldecossatun and travels via the lateral corticospinal tract to the anterior horn cells (ventral gray matter). Approximately 10% of fibers do not cross over in the medulla. They will travel in the ante-

rior corticspinal tracts to assist in voluntary motor control in the cervical and upper thoracic segments.

4. Upper motor neuron disorders

Cerebellar System

1. Responsible for:
   • Equilibrium
   • Posture control
   • Muscular activity
   • Sensory and motor input

2. Pathway varies: cortex or basal ganglia or sensory receptors; anterior horn cells

3. Lower motor neuron disorders

Extrapyramidal System

1. Responsible for:
   • Muscle tone
   • Control of body movements

2. Complex system of pathways between basal ganglia, brain stem, cerebral cortex, spinal cord, and anterior horn cells.

Chapter Four

Neurology

Disorders

Alzheimer's Disease

- A common degenerative disease that usually begins in later middle life with slight defects in memory and behavior.
- It occurs with equal frequency in men and women.
- The cerebral hemisphere undergoes marked atrophy with a widening of the sulci and lateral ventricles which can be seen on a C-scan.
- The disease is characterized by the patient's forgetfulness, paranoia, hostility, speech disturbances, confusion, and inability to carry out purposeful movements.
- Patient may become bedridden. It has no known cause, prevention, or cure.

Aneurysm

- A ballooning out of an arterial wall.
- It is usually caused by atherosclerosis and hypertension and less frequently by trauma, infection, or a congenital weakness in the vessel wall.
- Aneurysms most often occur in circle of Willis and are called berry aneurysms.

Anterior Cerebral Artery Lesion

- Contralateral hemiplegia
- Incontinence
- Hemiparesis

- Behavioral changes
- If this occurs in the nondominant hemisphere, apraxia would be indicated.
- If it occurs in the dominant hemisphere, aphasia would be indicated.

Anterior Communicating Artery Lesion

- Incontinence
- Impairment of intellect
- Innovative abilities lost
- Paraparesis

Anterior Inferior Cerebellar Artery Lesion

- Ipsilateral ataxia
- Contralateral pain and temperature deficits
- Ipsilateral deafness
- Ipsilateral facial paralysis
- Ipsilateral sensory loss to the face

Basal Ganglia Disorder

- **Parkinson's disease:** resting tremors, rigidity, shuffling gait, and mask-like face.
- **Chorea:** sudden uncontrolled movements; very jerky and brisk movements.
- **Athetosis:** very slow movements.
- **Hemiballismus:** sudden wild movements that involve only one side of the body.
- **Tremor:** an involuntary movement, usually with a consistent rhythm and amplitude.

Bell's Palsy

- Paralysis of the facial nerve.
- Typically occurs unilaterally and results in facial paralysis.
- It may be temporary or permanent.
- May result from infections, compression on a nerve by a tumor, or trauma to nerve.

Brown-Sequard Syndrome

- Hemisection of the spinal cord; may be seen after knife-type injury to the spinal cord.
- Ipsilateral lower motor neuron paralysis at lesion level.
- Ipsilateral upper motor neuron paralysis below lesion.
- Contralateral loss of pain/temperature below lesion.
- Ipsilateral loss of vibration and proprioception below lesion level.
- Ipsilateral loss of kinesthetic sense/muscle tone below lesion level.

Brain Tumors—Neoplasm

- Tumors are space-occupying lesions that produce edema and epileptic-like seizures.
- They may cause increased intracranial pressure, headache, and vomiting.
- Tumors of the cerebellum can cause ataxia and falling.
- Frontal pole tumors can cause personality changes or loss of smell.
- Pituitary edema can cause optical and visual disturbances.

Cerebellar Disorders

- **Ataxia:** person will have poor coordination, as well as posture and gait difficulties.
- **Athetosis:** slow, writhing, continuos involuntary movement of the extremities.
- **Chores:** involuntary muscle twitching.
- **Dysmetria:** when reaching for an object, the person will overshoot the goal/object.
- **Dysdiadochokinesia:** person will demonstrate an inability to perform alternating movements.
- **Asthenia:** person will get tired very easily.
- **Tremors:** rhythmic, involuntary, nonpurposefully movements.
- Decreased tendon reflexes
- Slurred speech

Cerebral Vascular Accidents

- May be defined as damage to the brain as a result of a pathological condition of the blood vessels.
- Characterized by occlusion by an embolus or cerebrovascular hemorrhage, which results in ischemia of the brain tissues normally perfused by the damaged vessels.

Encephalitis

- An inflammation of the brain.
- May be caused by an infected mosquito bite, poisoning, or hemorrhage.
- Characterized by fevers, headache, nausea, vomiting, and neck pain.
- Patient may demonstrates neurological disturbances, seizures, paralysis,weakness, and irritability.
- Severity of condition depends on many factors, such as age of patient, time of diagnosis, cause and level of inflammation.

Epilepsy

- Repeated seizures due to sudden uncontrolled electric discharge of the nerve cells of the cerebral cortex.
- Symptoms may include altered consciousness, convulsions, stiffness of muscles, movement spasticity of muscles.
- They can be petit mal seizures, which are brief, or grand mal seizures, which last 2 to 5 minutes.

Guillain-Barré Syndrome

- Peripheral polyneuritis (also called infectious polyneuritis).
- Associated with viral infections or immunizations.
- Results in symmetrical wasting away of the extremities.
- Course of disease varies in symptoms (from mild to severe) and length of recovery.

Hydrocephalus

- A blockage in the ventricular system.
- The cerebrospinal fluid is prevented from flowing out and instead accumulates in the ventricles. This increases pressure in the cranial vault and causes a thinning out of the brain and widening of the ventricles.
- Most often occurs in newborns in which cranial bones are not yet fused.
- The fluid separates the bone and the head enlarges.

Internal Carotid Artery Lesion

- Aphasia when in the dominant hemisphere
- Contralateral hemiplegia
- Hemianesthesia
- Hemianopia
- Unilateral loss of vision

Amyotrophic Lateral Sclerosis (Lou Gehrig's Disease)

- Amyotrophic lateral sclerosis
- Upper and lower motor neuron disease
- Sensory losses
  Ataxia
- Decreased muscle tone
- Loss of kinesthetic sense
- Progressive

Middle Cerebral Artery Lesion

A. Involves the **dominant side** main trunk of the middle cerebral artery
  - Motor aphasia
  - Sensory aphasia
  - Contralateral hemianesthesia
  - Hemiplegia
  - Homonymous hemianopsia

B. Involves the **nondominant side** main trunk of the middle cerebral artery
  - Denial of the disease
  - Contralateral hemiplegia
  - Contralateral hemianesthesia
  - Homonymous hemianopia
  - Neglect of the left side

C. This lesion occurs in the perforating branches of the artery
  - Contralateral hemiplegia
  - Contralateral rigidity
  - Tremor

Multiple Sclerosis

- Progressive disease resulting from demyelination of nerve fibers of the spinal cord or brain.
- It has periods of remission and exacerbation.
- Disease usually shows up in young adults.
- Results in ataxia, abnormal reflexes, paresthesia, muscle weakness, vertigo, and vision disturbance.
- Symptoms will vary and there is no known cure.

Myasthenia Gravis

- Result is a fluctuation of muscle strength/weakness, especially muscles of the eyelid, face, jaws, and limbs. As a result, the patient has a drooping jaw, difficulties with swallowing, speech, facial expression, and changing.
- Treatment: muscle strengthening, range of motion.

Parkinson's Disease

- A slow progressive degenerative neurologic disorder that usually affects people over 50 years of age.
- The disease is characterized by resting tremors, slow shuffling gait, forward flexion of the trunk, muscle rigidity and weakness, and a masklike face.
- It has no known cause, prevention, or cure.

Polio

- Involves damage to anterior horn cells
- Lower motor neuron involvement
- Weakness
- Atrophy
- Fasciculation
- Hyperflexion

Posterior Cerebral Artery Lesion

- The main trunk
- Contralateral hemiparesis
- Sensory aphasia—dominant side
- Hemianopia

- Loss of superficial touch
- Loss of deep sensation

Posterior Inferior Cerebral Artery Lesion

- Ataxia
- Contralateral hemianalgesia
- Difficulty swallowing
- Intentional tremors
- Ipsilateral weakness of the tongue
- Ipsilateral weakness of the vocal cords
- Nystagmus

Superior Cerebral Artery Lesion

- Contralateral hemianesthesia
- Contralateral hemianalgesia
- Contralateral facial weakness
- Ipsilateral ataxia

Transient Ischemic Attack (TIA)

- Defined as an episode of cerebrovascular insufficiency or occlusion of a small artery.
- This causes the patient to lose consciousness briefly, be confused and disoriented, experience difficulty with speech and tongue movement, but awake with no paralysis.
- The attack is usually brief, lasting a few minutes.

Upper Motor Neuron

- Spastic paralysis
- No muscle atrophy
- Hyperactive reflexes
- Pathological reflexes, Babinski sign
- Fasciculation/fibrillation not present

Lower Motor Neuron

- Flaccid paralysis
- Muscle atrophy
- Absent reflexes

- No pathological reflexes
- Fasciculation/fibrillation present

Vertebrobasilar Artery Lesion

- Anesthesia of both sides of the body
- Areflexia
- Coma
- Confusion/loss of memory
- Dizziness
- Headache

Neurology Diagnostic Test

Cerebral Angiography

An x-ray procedure for visualizing the vascular system of the brain. Radiopaque contract material is injected into a carotid, subclavian, brachial, or femoral artery with x-rays at specific intervals.

Computed Tomography (CT Scan)

An x-ray technique that produces a film representing a detailed cross-section of tissue structure. CT scan employs a narrowly collimated beam of x-rays that rotates in a continuous 360° motion around the patient. The image is created by computer, using multiple readings of the patient in cross-sectional slices. This is a noninvasive and painless procedure for the patient.

Echoencephalogram

A recording produced by an echoencephalograph, which uses ultrasound to study the intracranial structures of the brain.

Electroencephalography (EEG)

The process of recording brainwave activity. Electrodes are attached to various areas of the patient's head. The patient must refrain from talking or moving and must remain still. The test is used to diagnose seizure and brainstem disorders, focal lesions, and impaired consciousness.

Electromyogram (EMG)

A record of the intrinsic electric activity in a skeletal muscle is obtained by applying surface electrodes or by inserting a needle electrode into the muscle. The physician observes electric activity with an oscilloscope and a loudspeaker. EMGs also measure electric potentials induced by voluntary muscular contraction.

Evoked Potential (EP)

A tracing of a brainwave measured on the surface of the head at various places. The evoked potential is elicited by a specific stimulus that may affect the visual, somatosensory pathways, and auditory, producing a characteristic brainwave pattern.

Lumbar Puncture (LP)

The introduction of a hollow needle and stylet into the subarachnoid space of the lumbar portion of the spinal canal at the third and fourth lumbar vertebrae. The patient is placed in a lateral recumbent position, with the back as near the edge of the bed as possible. The legs should be flexed with the thighs flexed on the abdomen. Head and shoulders should be bent down, curving the spine convexly to grant the greatest amount of space between the vertebrae. The test is done to evaluate spinal fluid and measure intracranial pressure. The complications of testing may include headaches, infections, and epidural hematomas.

Magnetic Resonance Imaging (MRI)

Medical imaging that utilizes nuclear magnetic resonance as a source of energy. This procedure is noninvasive and painless for the patient. Allows for three-dimensional viewing and high resolution.

Myelography

A radiographic process by which the spinal cord and spinal subarachnoid space are viewed and photographed. A contrast medium is introduced. This test is used to identify spinal lesions.

Nerve Conduction Velocity (NCV)

Refers to the maximum nerve conduction velocity, which is the speed with which an electrical impulse can be transmitted through excitable tissue.

Position Emission Tomography (PET)

Radioisotopes are injected and emissions are measure by a gamma ray detector system.

This test does provide information on the cerebral blood flow and brain metabolism, however, its is not as detailed as computerized tomography or magnetic resonance imaging.

Ventriculography

An x-ray examination of the head after an injection of air or another contrast medium into the cerebral ventricles, or an x-ray examination of a ventricle of the heart after the injection of a radiopaque contrast medium.

Reflex

An involuntary response to a sensory stimulus.

Crossed Extension Reflex

Functions to coordinate reciprocal limb movement as in gait patterns.

Flexor Reflex

Functions as a protective withdrawal reflex to move the body away from a harmful stimulus.

Inverse Stretch Reflex

Functions to provide agonist inhibition and decreases the force of the agonist contraction.

Stretch Reflex

Functions to support agonist muscle contraction and maintenance of muscle tone by providing feedback about muscle length.

Grades of Muscle Stretch Reflexes

0	Areflexia
+	Hyporeflexia
1 to 3	Average
3+ to 4+	Hyperreflexia

Muscle Stretch Reflexes

Segmental and Nerve Level	Reflex	Stimulus	Response
Pons, trigeminal	Jaw maxillary nerve	Tap mandible, half open position	Closure of jaw
C5, C6 musculocutaneous nerve	Biceps	Tap biceps tendon	Contraction of biceps
C5, C6 musculocutaneous nerve	Brachioradialis	At insertion of brachio-radialis, styloid process of radius	Flexion of elbow and pronation of forearm
C5 to T1	Scapular, interscapular	Stroking skin between scapulae	Contraction of scapular muscles
C6, C7, C8 radial nerve	Triceps	Tap triceps tendon	Extension of elbow
C7, C8 radial nerve	Wrist extension	Tap wrist extensor tendons	Extension of wrist
C6, C7, C8 median nerve	Wrist flexion	Tap wrist flexor tendons	Flexion of wrist
L4, L5 superior gluteal nerve	Gluteal	Stroking skin of buttocks	Contraction of gluteus
L2, L3, L4 femoral nerve	Patellar	Tap patellar tendon	Extension of leg at knee
S1, S2 tibial nerve	Tendocalcaneus	Stroke Achilles' tendon	Plantar flexion at ankle
S1, S2 tibial nerve	Plantar	Stroke sole of foot	Plantar flexion of toes

Pathological Reflexes

Name	Stimulus	Response
Asymmetrical tonic reflex	Rotate the head to one side	Flexion of skull limbs and extension of jaw limbs
Babinski sign	Stroke the outer edge of the sole of the foot	Extension of great toe, flexion of small toes, and spreading of toes
Clonus—upper extremity	Rapid extension of wrist	Rapid reciprocal flexion and extension
Clonus—lower extremity	Rapid dorsiflexion of the ankle	Continued and prolonged reciprocal plantar flexion and dorsiflexion of the ankle
Cross extension	Patient supine, both legs flexed at hip, stimulate the sole of the foot	Extension of contralateral extremity
Extensor thrust	Therapist vigorously dorsiflexes the foot of a leg that has been flexed at hip	Extension of that entire lower extremity
Flexor withdrawal	Lower extremity in extended position stimulates sole of foot	The leg will withdraw from the stimulus; cause an over-response of hip and knee flexion
Forced grasping	Stroke the patient's palm in radial direction	Grasp reaction
Hirschberg's sign	Stroke the medial border of foot	Adduction and inversion of foot
Klippel-Weil thumb sign	Patient's flexed fingers are rapidly extended	Flexion and adduction of the thumb

Pathological Reflexes (Continued)

Name	Stimulus	Response
Marie-Fox	Forcefully flex the patient's toes	Flexion at hip and knee
Negative support reaction	Have patient bounce several times on soles of feet, but do not allow weightbearing	Flexor tone in lower extremities will increase
Positive support reaction	Have patient bounce several times on soles of feet, allowing the lower extremities to bear weight	Extensor tone in the lower extremities will increase
Righting reaction	Push the patient forward/backward and laterally	Head will try to orient itself, maintain midline
Rossolimo's sign	Tap on the balls of patient's foot	Flexion of toes
Strümpell's tibialis anterior sign	Patient flexes the hip	Dorsiflexion and adduction of the foot
Strümpell's pronation sign	Patient flexes the forearm	The hand touches the shoulder
Symmetrical tonic neck reflex	Place the head in flexion or extension	In flexed position, flexion of arms, extension of legs; with head extension, extension of arms, flexion of legs
Tonic labyrinthine	None required. Response depends on patient positioning	Prone: flexor tone increase. Supine: extensor tone increase. Sidelying: extensor tone in sidelying limbs will increase; flexor tone in nonweightbearing limbs will increase

Synergy Patterns

Synergy occurs as a result of the following:
- The muscles work together as one bound unit
- Reflexes occur at the spinal cord level
- The reflexes are primitive or automatic in nature

Upper Extremity

Joint	Flexion	Extension
Shoulder girdle	Elevation	Depression
	Retraction	Protraction
Shoulder	Abduction	*Adduction
	External rotation	Internal rotation
Elbow	*Flexion	Extension
Forearm	Supination	*Pronation
Wrist	Flexion	Extension
Fingers	Flexion	Flexion

Note: Wrist/fingers will vary

*Strong components of the synergism

Lower Extremity

Joint	Flexion	Extension
Hip	*Flexion	Extension
	*Abduction	*Adduction
	*External rotation	Internal rotation
Knee	Flexion	*Extension
Ankle	*Dorsiflexion	*Plantar flexion
Foot	Inversion	*Inversion
Toes	Dorsiflexion	Plantar flexion, great toe may extend

*Strong components of the synergism

Three Stages of Recovery in a CVA

1. Flaccid Stage
- Mobility in turning from supine to sidelying and sitting to supine
- Preparation for sitting up
- Preparation for standing up, control of leg
- Trunk balance
- Control of upper extremity
- Stimulation and facilitation to increase tone/voluntary movements

2. Spasticity
- Progression of treatment to work on rehabilitation of patient in the sitting and standing positions as much as possible. Some treatment started in stage 1 will still be performed in the supine position.
- Inhibition techniques to supine spasticity
- Weightbearing on extremity
- Sitting
- Standing
- Progression to treatment in prone lying and kneeling
- Gait training
- Working for independent control of extremity joints
- Facilitation for voluntary movement
- Placing

3. Stages of Relative Recovery
- Treatments to improve patient's gait, balance, and coordination
- Dissociation of mass patterns of movements
- Activities of daily living

Diagonal Patterns

PNF (proprioceptive neuromuscular facilitation) diagonals are named according to the movement that takes place. The pattern starts with the opposite positioning so that the maximal movement can take place. For example, D1 flexion for glenohumeral will start with the patient positioned in internal rotation, extension, and abduction. The finished position is then external rotation, flexion, and adduction.

Upper Extremity Diagonals

Diagonal One (D1)

Joint	Flexion	Extension
Scapula thoracic	Rotation, abduction, anterior elevation	Rotation, adduction, posterior depression
Glenohumeral	External rotation, flexion, adduction	Internal rotation, extension abduction
Elbow	Flexion	Extension
Radioulnar	Supination	Pronation
Wrist	Flexion, radial deviation	Extension, ulnar deviation
Fingers	Flexion, adduction to radial side	Extension, abduction to ulnar side
Thumb	Flexion, abduction	Extension, abduction

Diagonal Two (D2)

Joint	Flexion	Extension
Scapula thoracic	Rotation, abduction, posterior elevation	Rotation, abduction, anterior depression
Glenohumeral	External rotation, flexion, abduction	Internal rotation, extension, adduction
Elbow	Flexion	Extension
Radioulnar	Supination	Pronation
Wrist	Extension, radial deviation	Flexion, ulnar deviation
Finger	Extension, abduction to the radial side	Flexion, adduction to ulnar side
Thumb	Extension, adduction	Flexion, abduction

Lower Extremity Diagonals

Diagonal One (D1)

Joint	Flexion	Extension
Hip	External rotation, flexion, adduction	Internal rotation, extension, abduction
Knee	Flexion or extension	Extension or flexion
Ankle	Dorsiflexion	Plantar flexion
Subtalar	Inversion	Eversion
Toes	Extension, abduction to tibial side	Flexion, adduction to fibular side

Diagonal Two (D2)

Joint	Flexion	Extension
Hip	Internal rotation, flexion, abduction	External rotation, extension, adduction
Knee	Flexion or extension	Extension or flexion
Ankle	Dorsiflexion	Plantar flexion
Subtalar	Eversion	Inversion
Toes	Extension, abduction to the fibular side	Flexion, adduction to the tibial side

PNF Terms

Manual contact: firm contact over muscles facilitates the agonist to contract. Light touch may facilitate movement. Maintaining touch may facilitate a holding response. The therapist applies pressure (firm, light, or maintains pressure) for the purpose of stimulating the muscle, tendon, and joint afferent.

Maximal resistance: the therapist applies maximal resistance to stronger muscles in an attempt to create an overflow response to weaker muscles.

Reinforcement: the utilization of major muscle groups or other body parts coordinated to produce a desired movement pattern.

Timing for emphasis: maximum resistance in a sequence of contractions is used to elicit overflow from strong to weaker components. May be used for weakness or incoordination.

Traction: force used to separate a joint surface by manual contact.

PNF Techniques

Approximation: joint compression to stimulate afferent nerve endings. This is utilized to promote stability and facilitate postural extension.

Contract/relax: the therapist passively moves the body part to its limited point of range of motion. The patient then contracts the muscle against therapist resistance. The therapist resists all motion except for rotation. The patient then relaxes and the therapist moves it passively in the opposite direction caused by the contraction. This technique is used to increase range of motion of the agonist muscle.

Hold/relax: the therapist passively moves the body part to its limited point of range of motion. The patient contracts and the therapist provides resistance, allowing no movement to occur. This is different than contract/relax, in which rotation may occur. Next the patient is asked to relax allowing movement to take place and the therapist passively moves in the newly gained range of motion. Hold/relax is utilized to increase range of motion movement and decrease muscle spasms.

Repeated contractions: isometric contraction followed by repeated isotonic contraction and quick stretches. Can be performed anywhere within the patient's range of motion. Utilized to facilitate the agonist and relax the antagonist. It is performed on patients to increase strength, coordination, and endurance.

Rhythmic initiation: passive motion, then assistive motion, then resistive motion by alternating patterns to promote the ability to initiate movement, promotes relaxation, and decrease rigidity.

Rhythmic stabilization: performed by having the patient alternate isometric contraction of the agonist and antagonist muscles. Utilized to promote stability and to relax the antagonist.

Slow reversal: an alternating pattern of opposing muscle groups to stimulate the agonist through active motion, then relaxation of the antagonist, then coordination between agonist and antagonist. Utilized for a patient who has an inability to reverse direction and muscle imbalance. It will increase muscle strength, improve coordination, and increase endurance.

Slow reversal-hold: an alternating pattern of opposing muscle groups with a pause between reversals to cause relaxation of the antagonist and to stimulate the agonist. Utilized for a patient who has an inability to reverse direction and muscle imbalance. It will increase muscle strength, improve coordination, and increase endurance.

Slow reversal-hold-relax: the patient, through active range of motion, brings the body part to the point of limitation and then reverses direction. The therapist applies resistance to rotation and isometric contraction of the shortened muscle. Next, the patient relaxes and moves the body part in the direction of limitation. This technique is utilized repeatedly to increase range of motion of the agonist.

Berta Bobath Theory of Automatic Reactions

Berta Bobath, PT, and Karl Bobath, MD, developed this approach. Their treatment was based on the theory of inhibiting abnormal reflex patterns and facilitating righting and equilibrium reaction. The righting and equilibrium reactions are performed in a special sequential order according to development pattern to facilitate movement and control tone.

Three Automatic Reactions

Righting Reactions
- Maintain and restore normal position of the head in space.
- Maintain and restore normal position of the head with regard to trunk alignment.
- Maintain and restore normal position of the head and the four extremities.
- Align the body as necessary for various motor activities.
- Overlap with equilibrium reactions.
- Adjust posture.

Equilibrium Reactions
- Automatic reactions that maintain and restore balance during activities.
- Inhibition of abnormal patterns of posture and movement.

Automatic Adaptation of Muscle Joints to Changes in Posture
- Postural reflex mechanisms
- Postural adaptation to growth
- Assessment
  - ✓ Balance

- ✓ Range of motion
- ✓ Postural tone
- ✓ Motor patterns (quality of movement)
- ✓ Sensory deficit—pressure/light touch
- ✓ Proprioception
- ✓ Stereognosis
- ✓ Postural reactions
- ✓ Placing
- Emphasis on the quality of movement available, postural and protective reactions, and postural tone.

Signe Brunnstrom's Theory of Rehabilitation For a CVA

Brunnstrom, unlike Berta Bobath, believed that you should enhance the synergy patterns for treatment. Signe Brunnstrom's theory describes six stages of recovery for the hemiplegic patient. They are:

1. **Initial stage:** no voluntary movement of the affected limb can be initiated; spasticity is absent. Through evaluation, no voluntary movements are present, little or no resistance to passive movements.

2. **Recovery stage:** basic limb synergies are now appearing as weak associated reactions on voluntary attempts to move by the patient. The basic limb synergies in their components now make their appearance as weak associated reactions. This is where you start to see the beginning of flexor synergy patterns of the upper extremity and extensor synergy patterns of the lower extremity. Evaluation of the patient will demonstrate that when movement is attempted there is associated movements through synergy patterns.

3. **Stage three:** the basic limb synergies are performed voluntarily by the patient. In this stage spasticity is also increasing. Upon evaluation, there is full upper extremity synergy patterns along with ankle flexion.

4. **Stage four:** the patient progressed beyond stage three and the spasticity begins to decrease. Here you might observe some initial movement combinations that deviate from the basic limb synergy

patterns. The patient may have lateral prehension and semivoluntary finger extension. Upon evaluation, the patient can place his or her hand behind the back, flex the glenohumeral joint with elbow extension, pronate and supinate the forearm with elbow flexion at 90°, sit and dorsiflex the foot while keeping the foot on the floor, sit and slide the foot on the floor by flexing the knee past 90°.

5. **Stage five:** spasticity continues to decrease and the patient increasingly becomes independent from the basic limb synergies. The patient has palmar prehension and voluntary extension of digits. Upon evaluation the patient can perform the test in stage four with greater ease and efficiency. He or she can abduct at the glenohumeral joint with elbow extended, flex the shoulder past 90° with elbow extended, pronate/supinate the forearm with elbow extension and abduction of glenohumeral joint, stand nonweightbearing with effected limb, knee flexed and hip extended, stand with heel forward, knee extended, and dorsiflex the ankle.

6. **Stage six:** patient demonstrates isolated joint movements that are now freely performed. Movements appear to be well coordinated and near normal. The basic limb synergies no longer interfere with the patient's movement. Upon evaluation, the patient can perform the test in stage five with greater ease and efficiency. The patient can stand and abduct the hip, sit and reciprocally contract the medial and lateral hamstring muscles, causing inversion and eversion.

Brunnstrom's Stages of Recovery for the Upper Extremity

1. **Stage one:** initially, the upper extremity is flaccid and no voluntary movement on the affected limb can be initiated.

2. **Stage two:** the beginning of spasticity. Basic limb synergies or some other components are present.

3. **Stage three:** the active initiation of synergies. Spasticity has increased and becomes marked.

4. **Stage four:** patient's movement deviates from the synergies. Example: patient has elevation of the arm to forward horizontal

position with the elbow fully extended. Movement deviating from the synergy would be stage four. There are some movement combinations that deviate from the basic limb synergies.

5. **Stage five:** patient performs movement independent of the synergy. Spasticity is decreasing. Example: patient can abduct the arm to the side position with the elbow fully extended and the forearm pronated.

6. **Stage six:** isolate joint movement. Movements are well coordinated and appear normal. Example: patient would have lateral prehension for grasping small objects, such as a card.

Brunnstrom's Stages of Recovery for the Lower Extremity

1. **Stage one:** flaccidity.

2. **Stage two:** minimal voluntary movements of the lower limb.

3. **Stage three:** the ability to perform hip-knee-ankle flexion in sitting.

4. **Stage four:** the ability to perform voluntary dorsiflexion of the ankle in sitting.

5. **Stage five:** the ability to stand isolated, nonweightbearing with knee flexion and hip extended.

6. **Stage six:** the ability to stand and perform outward rotation of the leg at the knee, as well as inversion and eversion of the ankle.

Brunnstrom's Stages of Recovery for the Hand

1. **Stage one:** flaccidity.

2. **Stage two:** no active finger flexion.

3. **Stage three:** mass grasp.

4. **Stage four:** lateral prehension.

5. **Stage five:** palmar prehension.

6. **Stage six:** control of all prehension.

Brunnstrom Evaluates the Quality of Movement as Follows

- Nonfunctional (NF)
- Assistive (A)
- Functional (F)

The therapist is instructed to select a grade (NF, A, or F) for movement of the upper extremity, lower extremity, and trunk.

Rood Sensory Stimulation Techniques

Theory by Margaret Rood, who was a physical therapist and occupational therapist.

Basic Principles

1. Motor output is dependent upon sensory input. Therefore, you can use sensory stimulus to activate and inhibit a motor response.

2. Motor response follows a normal developmental sequence pattern. Stages of muscle development:
   - Full range of shortening and lengthening and reciprocal innervation
   - Patterns of cocontraction and stability; tonic postural set
   - Patterns of heavy weight movement and movement in weight-bearing position
   - Skilled or coordinated movement; movement in nonweight-bearing position with stabilization at proximal joint

3. In early stages, patients who do not demonstrate motor control would benefit from sensory stimulus.

4. Early use of stimulus should be discontinued as soon as patient demonstrates active control. This decreases dependence upon the therapist.

5. Patients who show a low-level response to stimulus may need repeated application of stimulus or a combination of stimulus to produce results.

6. Avoid overloading a patient with too much sensory stimulation and causing an overload effect.

Stimulation Techniques

Exteroceptive Stimulation Techniques

- High-frequency vibration (50 to 300 Hz): facilitation of agonist, inhibition of antagonist.
- Low-frequency vibration (5 to 50 Hz): inhibition of agonist.
- Neutral warmth (35° to 37°C): relaxation, inhibition of postural tone, decreased pain, calming effect.
- Pressure on tendons: firm, constant pressure to decreased tone, and generalized inhibition.
- Prolonged icing: inhibition of muscle tone, spasms, and pain.
- Quick icing facilitation of muscles.
- Quick stretch, tapping of muscle belly or tendon: facilitation of agonist.
- Prolonged stretch: inhibition of muscle response or decrease of tone.

Vestibular Stimulation Techniques

- Fast spinning: facilitates postural tone, promotes head righting and increased motor coordination.
- Head down position, prone over a large ball: can activate postural extensors of neck, trunk, and proximal joints. Soothing effect, especially sympathetic responses.
- Slow rocking, rolling on ball: inhibits postural tone; calming effect and relaxation.

Proprioception Stimulation Techniques

- Quick stretch
- Tapping of muscle belly or tendon
- Joint approximation
- Joint traction
- High-frequency vibration
- Low-frequency vibration
- Prolonged slow stretch
- Firm pressure to tendons

Levels of Cognitive Function

Ranchos Los Amigos Scale

1. Level one—No response.
   Patient is unresponsive to any stimulus and appears to be in a deep sleep.

2. Level two—Generalized response.
   Patient occasionally reacts to stimuli but not in a purposeful pattern. Response is limited and inconsistent.

3. Level three—Localized response.
   Patient reacts to stimuli but continues to be inconsistent. May follow simple commands in a delayed manner.

4. Level four—Confused/agitated.
   Patient responds to stimuli but is unable to process information purposefully. Patient is in a heightened state of activity and behavior is bizarre. Patient is not able to cooperate with treatment program.

5. Level five—Confused/inappropriate/nonagitated.
   Patient is alert and able to follow very simple commands with fluctuating consistency. If instructions are increasing in complexity, the patient will demonstrate inconsistency.

6. Level six—Confused/appropriate.
   Patient can follow directions but only with direct assistance from another individual. Goal-oriented behavior with directions.

7. Level Seven—Automatic/appropriate.
   Patient can go through daily routine automatically but robot-like, with shallow recall of activities.

8. Level eight—Purposeful/appropriate.
   Patient shows carryover for new learning and needs no supervision once activities are learned. Patient is able to recall and is aware of and responsive to environment.

Level of Consciousness

Glasgow Coma Scale

- This scale is utilized to determine the level of consciousness of the patient.
- The patient is scored according to three categories:
  1. Eye opening
  2. Verbal response
  3. Motor response

- The test is administered and the score added. If the patient has a score of 9 or above, he or she is determined not clinically diagnosed to be in a coma. A score of 7 or less would indicate that the patient is in a coma.

Glasgow Coma Scale

Eye Opening
Spontaneous: 4 points
Indicates that brain arousal systems are active.

To sound: 3 points
Eyes will open to sound stimulus

To pain: 2 points
Eyes will open to pain stimulus applied to extremities

Never: 1 point

Motor Response
Obeys commands: 6 points
May not have a grasp reflex or a change in posture as a response

Localized: 5 points
Will attempt to respond to stimulus by moving extremity

Flexor normal: 4 points
In response to stimulus, will flex entire shoulder or arm

Flexion abnormal: 3 points
Response to painful stimulus is decorticating rigidity posture

Extension: 2 points
Response is abnormal adduction with internal rotation of the shoulder and pronation of the forearm

None: 1 point

Verbal Response
Oriented: 5 points
Patient will know who, where they are, month, year, and season

Confused: 4 points
Responds to questions but will have some degree of confusion and disorientation

Inappropriate: 3 points
Speech is understandable but patient cannot sustain a conversation

Incomprehensible: 2 points
Speech is not understandable but patient can make sounds of moaning and groans

None: 1 point

Neurological Assessment

1. History
2. Patient interview
3. Vital signs
4. Motor function:
    a. Strength
    b. Atrophy
    c. Fatigue
    d. Muscle tone
    e. Motor control
5. Sensory function:
    a. Protective sensations
    b. Discriminative sensation
    c. Sensory deficits
6. Activities of daily living
7. Functional mobility skills
8. Speech/communication abilities
9. Gait/transfers
10. Posture
    a. General posture: posterior and side views
    b. Postural synergies
11. Respiratory system
12. Balance
    a. Standing: single limb and double limb support
    b. Dynamic: walking, turning, bending
    c. Rhomberg test
13. Coordination
    a. Equilibrium
    b. Nonequilibrium
14. Cognitive/behavioral status
15. Vision
16. Skin integrity
17. Endurance/fatigue levels
18. Pain

Chapter Five
Cranial Nerve Assessment

Cranial Nerve I: Olfactory

Function

Smell

Test

Ask the patient to identify different smells with his or her eyes closed.

Cranial Nerve II: Optic

Function

Vision

Test

Ask the patient to close one eye while you move a finger in sight of the patient, then away, asking the patient to report when it is out of his or her vision.

Cranial Nerve III: Oculomotor

Function

Eye movements

Test

Ask the patient to perform the following: elevation and depression of the eye. Assess quality of eye movements and note any deviations.

Cranial Nerve IV: Trochlear

Function

Eye movements

Test

Ask the patient to perform adduction and depression of the eye. Assess quality of movement and note deviations in eye movements.

Cranial Nerve V: Trigeminal

Function

Sensation of the face and scalp

Test

Test the patient's corneal reflex by gently touching the cornea with cotton. Ask the patient to close or clench the jaw and hold against resistance.

Cranial Nerve VI: Abducens

Function

Eye movements

Test

Ask the patient to abduct the eye and note movement.

Cranial Nerve VII: Facial

Function

- Taste, facial expressions, secretion of saliva and tears
- Pain and temperature of the external auditory meatus

Test

Evaluate the patient's taste by placing salt, sugar, or vinegar in small amounts on the tongue and see if he or she can identify the taste. Be sure to have the patient clear tastes in between tests by sipping water. Ask the patient to wrinkle the forehead or close the eyes against pressure.

Cranial Nerve VIII: Vestibulocochlear

Function

Hearing and balance/postural responses

Test

Take a ticking watch or timer and move it away from patient's ear. Have the patient tell you when he or she can no longer hear the ticking. Test both ears and note distance. Test the patient utilizing the finger-to-therapist's finger test.

Cranial Nerve IX: Glossopharyngeal

Function

- Sensation to the posterior one-third of the tongue
- Innervation of the stylopharyngeus muscle

Test

Assess taste to the posterior one-third of the tongue utilizing stimuli such as salt, sugar, or vinegar.

Cranial Nerve X: Vagus

Function

Swallowing, articulation, gag reflex

Test

Ask the patient to swallow and observe. Test the gag reflex. Ask the patient to say "hi" and observe articulation.

Cranial Nerve XI: Spinal Accessory

Function

Muscles of the pharynx, soft palate, and neck movements

Test

Ask the patient to shrug his or her shoulders while the therapist applies resistance.

Cranial Nerve XII: Hypoglossal

Function

Movement of the tongue

Test

Ask the patient to protrude the tongue and observe for deviations in movement.

Chapter Six

Spinal Cord

Types of Spinal Cord Injuries

Anterior Cord Syndrome

Results in damage to the anterior part of the spinal cord. This is an incomplete lesion and sense of light touch, proprioception, and position are usually intact. Bilateral loss of motor function, sensation of pain, and temperature. Typically caused by an injury that causes the loss of function from the anterior spinal artery.

Brown-Sequard Syndrome

Results in hemisection of the spinal cord. Typically seen after a stab wound or gunshot injury. This is also an incomplete lesion, which typically results in loss of motor function on the same side as the lesion and loss of pain and temperature on the opposite side. It is rare to have a complete hemisection on one side of the spinal cord; it is more likely the patient will have an irregular lesion. Lateral column damage will result in a positive Babinski sign and a loss of proprioception in the dorsal column, vibratory, and kinesthesia senses.

Cauda Equina Injury

Involves the lower end of the spinal cord at the first lumbar vertebra and the bundle of lumbar, sacral, and coccygeal nerve roots that emerge from the spinal cord and descend through the spinal canal of the sacrum and coccyx before reaching the intervertebral foramina of their particular vertebrae.

Central Cord Syndrome

Occurs when there is damage to the central portion of the cord and is an incomplete lesion. Typically greater deficits are found in the upper extremities than in the lower extremities upon evaluation. Hyperextension injuries of the cervical spine typically cause the central cord syndrome.

Complete Lesion

Occurs when the entire spinal cord is severed. It results in no sensation or muscle power below the level of the lesion. Complete lesion is usually the result of severe compression, extensive vascular dysfunction, and transection.

Discomplete Lesion

Signifies that the spinal cord is partially injured, but discomplete. It results from sparing of a small amount of axons in the spinal cord.

Incomplete Lesion

A partial loss of sensation or voluntary muscle power below the neurological level of the lesion. Incomplete lesions are usually the result of edema in the spinal cord and bony protrusion or bone fragments in the spinal cord.

Paraplegia

Injury classification for patients who loose function of both lower extremities. Typically, the injury level is between T1 and L1.

Posterior Cord Syndrome

This is a rare syndrome and typically not seen in spinal cord injuries. It will result in loss of proprioception and a steppage gait. The loss is below the level of the lesion.

Quadriplegia

Injury classification for patients who loose function of all four extremities and trunk. The injury level is between C1 and C8.

Sacral Sparing

Occurs in the sacral area and is an incomplete lesion. Typically, sensation will be intact in the sacral area; however, paralysis and loss of sensation are complete in all other areas below the level of lesion.

Spinal Cord Impairment/Classification Scales

American Spinal Injury Association Impairment Scale

Grade A: Complete lesion, no sensory or motor function is intact in the S4 to S5 segment level.

Grade B: Incomplete lesion, sensory but no motor function below neurological level. Sensory function is intact through S4 to S5.

Grade C: Incomplete lesion, motor function is intact below the neurological level. Most key muscles below the level have a muscle grade of less then three.

Grade D: Incomplete lesion, motor function is intact below the neurological level. Most key muscles below the level have a muscle grade of three or more.

Grade E: Normal sensory and motor function.

Modified Frankel Classification Scale

Grade A: Complete sensory and motor involvement.

Grade B: Complete motor involvement and some sensory sparing.

Grade C: Motor sparing but is not functional.

Grade D: Motor sparing that is functional.

Grade E: No neurological involvement.

Medical Complications of a Spinal Cord Injury

Autonomic Hyperreflexia

- A distended bladder, distended rectum, or neurological procedures with catheterizations or bladder irrigation generally cause this. This condition can occur in any patient with a lesion above the T5 level.
- Symptoms may include pounding headache, hypertension, sweating above the level of the spinal cord injury, slow pulse, and nasal obstruction.

- The therapist should monitor symptoms. If the above symptoms are seen, the patient should be positioned in sitting immediately to create postural hypotension or decrease the blood pressure. This can be performed only if the patient's spine is stable enough for him or her to be in the sitting position. The therapist should check the catheter and tubing, empty the leg bag if it is full and, depending upon the severity of the symptoms, notify the attending physician or nurse.

Bowel and Bladder Complications

- Urination is controlled by the conus medullaris, and primary reflex control is in the sacral segments.
- Spinal shock and lesions above the conus medullaris result in the bladder being flaccid, absent reflexes, a reflex neurogenic bladder, and reflex bowel. This will result in spasticity, ureteral reflux, voiding complications, and detrusor muscle hypertrophy.
- Lesions at the conus medullaris result in the bladder being nonreflexive, decreased tone of the ureteral sphincter and perineal muscles, and nonreflex bowel.

Heterotopic Ossification

- This is defined as ectopic or hypertrophic bone growth. It is an abnormal occurrence of bone growth in the soft tissue, usually the tendons and connective tissue. Typically, the hip, knee, elbow, and shoulder joints are most frequently involved. The specific cause is unknown, although it appears frequently in spinal cord population, predominantly in males, and unilaterally or bilaterally in the hips. Heterotopic ossification occurs within the first year of injury and below the level of the lesion.
- Symptoms include pain, warmth, and edema.
- Treatment includes stretching and range of motion exercises.

Ulcers or Pressure Sores

- Caused by improper pressure relief or breakdown of the skin and tissue.
- Symptoms may include redness or red spots, and/or skin breakdown.
- Treatment includes teaching the patient the proper pressure relief. The patient needs to be able to relieve ischial pressure, sacral pressure, and greater trochanter pressure. The patient needs to learn weight shifting, independent pressure relief, and repositioning.

Methods of Bracing/Stabilizing a Spinal Cord Injury

Foot Orthosis (AFO)

A short leg brace designed to prevent the patient from tripping secondary to weak or absent dorsiflexors. This is an L-shaped brace typically made out of plastic.

Halo

An external brace designed to stabilize the cervical vertebrae.

Harrington Rods

Rods placed internally to stabilize either the thoracic or lumbar vertebrae.

Jewett Orthosis

An external method of providing stabilization to the thoracic and lumbar vertebrae. This is a three-point brace that prevents hyperextension, with the three points of pressure on the sternum, lumbar spine, and synthesis pubis.

Knee-Ankle-Foot-Orthosis (KAFO)

A long leg brace that stabilizes the knee and ankle. Brace may be metal or plastic.

Knight-Taylor Orthosis

A method of applying external stabilization to the thoracic and lumbar vertebrae. Typically utilized for fractures above the L3 region.

Scott-Craig Orthosis

A metal KAFO used by spinal cord patients.

Sterno-Occipital Mandibular Immobilization (SOMI)

A method of external stabilization for the cervical vertebrae.

Thoracic-Lumbar-Sacral Orthosis (TLSO)

Any orthosis that provides external immobilization of the thoracic and lumbar spine.

Weiss Springs

An internal stabilization method for the thoracic and lumbar vertebrae.

Common Muscle Substitutions

The spinal cord patient will use muscle substitution in areas where voluntary muscle activity may not be present or only partially available. Following is the muscle and its typical substitution.

Muscle	Substitutions
Upper trapezius	Levator scapulae
Middle trapezius	Rhomboids, levator scapulae
Rhomboids	Middle trapezius
Serratus anterior	Pectoralis minor and coracobrachialis
Biceps	Brachioradialis
Pectoralis major	Long head of the biceps, anterior deltoid
Triceps	Supraspinatus, infraspinatus, teres minor
Deltoid	Long head of the biceps, long head of the triceps, supraspinatus, infraspinatus, and teres minor
Supinator	Biceps, brachioradialis, external rotators of the shoulder, extensor muscles of the wrist, and supinator muscles of the forearm
Shoulder—external rotator	Supinators of the forearm and extensors of the wrist to rotate the arm with gravity
Shoulder—internal rotator	Pectoralis minor and coracobrachialis
Wrist extensors	Supination of the forearm or externally rotating the shoulder so gravity can extend the wrist
Wrist flexors	Pronating the forearm or internally rotating the shoulder so gravity can flex the wrist

Muscle	Substitutions
Pronators	Brachioradialis
Latissimus dorsi	Teres major, posterior deltoid, lower trapezius
Abdominals	Neck flexors, pectoralis major and minor, and serratus anterior
Quadrantus lumborum	Latissimus dorsi
Oblique abdominal	Latissimus dorsi
Hip flexors	Lower abdominal muscles
Hip extensors	Lower back extensor muscles
Hip abductors	Latissimus dorsi
Hip adductors	Lower abdominal muscles
Hip internal rotators	Lower abdominal muscles
Hip external rotators	Lower back extensors
Knee flexors	Sartorius and gracilis
Quadriceps	Adductor magnus
Inversion of the foot	Medial gastrocnemius
Eversion of the foot	Lateral gastrocnemius

Expected Functional Outcome of Spinal Cord Injuries According to Level

Cervical Spine Injuries

C1, C2, C3 Spinal Cord Injury

- Respiration: dependence on a respirator, may use phrenic nerve stimulator during the day.
- Bed mobility: needs a full-time attendant.
- Pressure relief: electric wheelchair with recline backs, dependent.
- Transfers: dependence on caregiver.
- Mobility in the wheelchair: electric wheelchair with sip and puff control may be utilized, seat belt, and trunk support.

C4 Spinal Cord Injury

- Respiration: vital capacity of at least 30% to 50% of the norm.
- Bed mobility: patient is able to direct bed mobility and give occasional minimal assistance.

- Pressure relief: patient is able to direct pressure relief activities or utilize reclining back on wheelchair.
- Transfers: patient is able to direct all transfers, otherwise dependent.
- Mobility in the wheelchair: patient is independent using a motorized wheelchair without hand controls on level surfaces, use breath, sip and puff, chin, or mouth controls.

C5 Spinal Cord Injury
- Respiration: vital capacity of 40% to 60% of norm; patient can assist with bronchial hygiene.
- Bed mobility: patient can give minimal assistance, overhead swivel bar.
- Pressure relief: patient may assist in changing wheelchair position, recline back—otherwise dependent.
- Transfers: patient is able to direct transfers, as well as give minimal assistance, overhead swivel bar, sliding board.
- Mobility in the wheelchair: patient is independent utilizing a motorized wheelchair with hand controls or electric wheelchair with joystick or adopted upper extremity controls.

C6 Spinal Cord Injury
- Respiration: vital capacity of 60% to 80% of norm; possibly independent with bronchial hygiene.
- Bed mobility: independent with side rails.
- Pressure relief: independent.
- Transfers: independent to and from a level surface, patient could give moderate assistance in all transfers, sliding board.
- Mobility in the wheelchair: independent with a manual wheelchair on level surfaces.
- Range of motion: patient is independent.

C7 Spinal Cord Injury
- Respiration: vital capacity of 60% to 80% of norm; independent with bronchial hygiene.
- Bed mobility: independent without special equipment.
- Pressure relief: independent, including wheelchair push-ups.
- Transfers: patient is able to give moderate assistance with transfers to and from the wheelchair and be independent on all level surfaces.

- Mobility in the wheelchair: patient is independent on level surfaces and able to assist on elevation.
- Range of motion: patient is independent.

C8 to T1 Spinal Cord Injury
- Respiration: vital capacity of 60-80% of norm; independent with bronchial hygiene.
- Bed mobility: patient is independent without special equipment.
- Pressure relief: patient is independent, including wheelchair push-ups.
- Transfers: patient is able to give moderate assistance with transfers to and from wheelchair.
- Mobility in the wheelchair: patient is independent on a level surface and able to assist on elevation.
- Range of motion: patient is independent.

Thoracic Spine Injuries

T1 to T5 Spinal Cord Injury
- Respiration: vital capacity of 80% of norm.
- Bed mobility: independent without special equipment.
- Pressure relief: independent, including wheelchair push-ups.
- Transfers: independent to and from the floor.
- Mobility in the wheelchair: independent in a manual wheelchair on all-level surfaces and elevations.
- Ambulation: it might be possible for the patient to be independent with bilateral KAFO and the parallel bars.
- Range of motion: independent.

T6 to T8 Spinal Cord Injury
- Respiration: vital capacity of 80% of norm.
- Bed mobility: independent without special equipment.
- Pressure relief: independent, including wheelchair push-ups.
- Transfers: independent to and from the floor.
- Mobility in the wheelchair: independent in a manual wheelchair on all level surfaces.
- Ambulation: supervision with bilateral KAFO and a walker; it might be possible for the patient to be independent with bilateral KAFO and a walker.
- Range of motion: independent.

T9 to T11 spinal cord Injury

- Respiration: vital capacity of 80% of norm.
- Bed mobility: independent without special equipment.
- Pressure relief: independent, including wheelchair push-ups.
- Transfers: independent to and from the floor.
- Ambulation: patient is able to use bilateral KAFO and Lofstrand crutches with supervision on elevations and rough terrain.
- Range of motion: independent.

T12 Spinal Cord Injury

- Respiration: vital capacity of 80% of norm.
- Bed mobility: independent without special equipment.
- Pressure relief: independent, including wheelchair push-ups.
- Transfers: independent to and from the floor.
- Ambulation: possible for patient to be independent with bilateral KAFO and Lofstrand crutches on all surfaces.
- Range of motion: independent.

Lumbar Spine Injuries

L1 to L3 Spinal Cord Injury

- Respiration: vital capacity of 80% of norm.
- Bed mobility: independent without special equipment.
- Pressure relief: independent, including wheelchair push-ups.
- Transfers: independent to and from the floor.
- Mobility in the wheelchair: independent in a manual wheelchair on all level surfaces.
- Ambulation: independent with bilateral KAFO and Lofstrand crutches on all surfaces.
- Range of motion: independent.

L4 to L5 Spinal Cord Injury

- Respiration: vital capacity of 80% of norm.
- Bed mobility: independent without special equipment.
- Pressure relief: independent, including wheelchair push-ups.
- Transfers: independent to and from the floor, independent on all level surfaces.
- Mobility in the wheelchair: independent in a manual wheelchair on all-level surfaces and elevations.
- Ambulation: independent with bilateral KAFO and crutches or canes.
- Range of motion: independent.

Level, Key Muscles, and Available Movements

This chart shows several key muscles and available movements at the neurological level where they add functional outcomes in the patient.

Level	Key Muscles	Available Movements
C1 to C3	Face and neck muscles: cranial innervation	Talking, sipping, blowing
C4	Diaphragm, trapezius	Scapular elevation, respiration
C5	Biceps, brachialis, brachioradialis, deltoid, infraspinatus, rhomboid major, rhomboid minor, supinator	Elbow flexion and supination, shoulder external rotation, shoulder abduction to 90°, limited shoulder flexion
C6	Extensor carpi radialis, infraspinatus, latissimus dorsi, pectoralis major, pronator teres, serratus anterior, teres minor	Shoulder flexion, extension, internal rotation and adduction, scapular abduction and upward rotation, forearm pronation, wrist extension
C7	Extensor pollicus longus and brevis, extrinsic finger flexion, flexor carpi radialis, triceps	Elbow extension, wrist flexion, finger extension
C8 to T1	Extrinsic finger flexors, flexor carpi ulnaris, flexor pollicis longus, flexor pollicis brevis, intrinsic finger flexor	Full innervation of upper extremity muscles
T4 to T6	Top half of intercostals, sacrospinalis and semispinalis (long muscles of the back)	Improve trunk control, increase respiratory reserve
T9 to T12	Lower abdominals, all intercostals	Improve trunk control, increase endurance

Level	Key Muscles	Available Movements
L2 to L4	Gracilis, iliopsoas, quadratus lumborum, rectus femoris, sartorius	Hip flexion, hip adduction, knee extension
L4, L5	Extensor digitorum, low back muscles, medial hamstrings, posterior tibialis, quadriceps, tibialis anterior	Strong hip flexion, strong knee extension, weak knee flexion, improve trunk control

Assessment

- **Patient interview:** interview the patient for medical history, history of injury, support medications, patient goals, and overall health.
- **Patient's skin:** pressure sores, redness, blisters, and any type of skin breakdown.
- **Vital signs:** blood pressure, respiratory rate, and heart rate in all positions.
- **Sensory:** pain, temperature, light touch, and proprioception.
- **Home safety:** home assessment for safety considerations and modifications.
- **Exercise:** exercise level of patient prior to injury and available level now.
- **Cognitive functioning:** patient's current mental status and processing abilities.
- **Musculoskeletal:** assess the patient's ability for motor planning, mobility, muscular strength, and endurance.
- **Respiration:** patient's color, breathing pattern, cough, and chest exam; utilization of respiratory muscles and diaphragm; presence of artificial airways.
- **Range of motion:** active or passive range of motion; complete evaluation of all motion available at each joint.
- **Muscle tone:** quality of the muscle tone—mild, moderate, or severe increase. Does the tone fluctuate?
- **Balance:** protective reactions, as well as equilibrium reactions.
- **Tolerance to vertical position:** can the patient tolerate vertical position in standing or sitting, any medical complication with vertical positioning?

- **Coordination:** kinesthetic awareness, timing, and accuracy of movement.
- **ADL activities:** activities of daily living, patient's possibility of becoming independent.
- **Social support:** family support and significant others.
- **Posture:** look at posture of patient and evaluate preventing contractures.
- **Gait:** is gait possible? What type of adaptive devices and patient goals for gait?

Treatment Options

- **Range of motion:** teach patient self range of motion when injury level allows, positioning to prevent contractures, and self-stretching. Teach patient and family orsupport personnel to carry over program to home.
- **Strengthening of available movements:** strengthen muscles that are still innervated and provide resistant exercise over time for strengthening and preventing atrophy.
- **Prevention teaching to patient and support system:** teach the patient and support system range of motion exercises, skin inspections, and home safety considerations.
- **Respiratory:** teach bronchial hygiene, assistive coughing, improve respiratory capacity, and breathing exercises.
- **Activities of daily living (ADLs):** assist the patient in performing as many activities of living independently as possible by level of lesion. Teach adaptive devices and fitting for assistance in ADLs.
- **Postural control:** teach proper posture with emphasis on stretching of hamstrings to maintain length. Hamstring length is necessary for transfer, standing, and gait. Correct posture will also assist with pain relief from muscular tightness that may develop.
- **Wheelchair mobility:** assist patients with fitting of wheelchair, wheelchair adjustments, promote wheelchair independence, teach wheelchair independence in all conditions—outdoors and inside. Teach transfers in and out, emergency techniques, and how to get back in a wheelchair in case of falls.
- **Pressure relief:** teach the patient and support system pressure relief techniques.

- **Stability:** teach the patient static balance and control. For example, apply resistance to the head to encourage shoulder stabilization.
- **Orthotic prescriptions:** assist the patient in ordering, fitting, and instructions for orthotics.
- **Cardiovascular endurance:** improve cardiovascular endurance, upper extremity ergonometery and swimming when possible.
- **Transfers:** teach the patient transfer to all surfaces—in and out of cars and bed. Teach patient how to utilize assistive devices for transfer (eg, transfer on sliding boards).
- **Ambulation:** work with the patient toward the goal of ambulation when possible, start with standing tolerance, first supported then unsupported. Functional electrical stimulation can be utilized to stimulate muscles.
- **Support groups:** assist the patient with emotional support when possible and give the patient information on support groups.
- **Referral to other services:** when necessary, facilitate referrals to other services to promote a team approach to the patient's treatment program.

Chapter Seven
Cardiac Anatomy & Physiology

Blood Supply

Arteries

Transport oxygenated blood to the heart through the heart pump to maintain arterial circulation.

Right Coronary Artery

Supplies the right atrium, most of the right ventricle, inferior wall of the left ventricle in most humans; bundle of His, atrioventricular node, and sinoatrial node in approximately 60% of humans.

Left Main Coronary Artery

Supplies most of the left ventricle mass and splits into two branches: the circumflex artery and left anterior descending artery. The circumflex artery supplies the inferior wall of the left ventricle when not supplied by the right coronary artery, left atrium, and sinoatrial node in approximately 40% of humans. The left anterior descending artery supplies the left ventricle, interventricular septum, right ventricle, and inferior areas of the apex and both ventricles.

Coronary Artery Dominance

The right coronary artery is dominant in approximately two-thirds of humans and branches into the posterior descending branches. The right coronary artery will supply part of the left ventricle and ventricular septum. This is called "right dominance." In one-third of humans the branch of the circumflex artery is dominant. Dominance is from branches of both the right coronary artery and the circumflex artery. This is called left dominance.

Capillaries

These are tiny blood vessels that assist in exchange of nutrients and fluids between the blood and tissue. In the heart, they connect the arteries to the veins, creating a large network system.

Veins

These transport unoxygenated blood from the whole body (except the lungs) to the right atrium of the heart. The coronary sinus drains the left atrium and both ventricles and the posterior right atrium and ventricles. The anterior cardiac vein drains the anterior right ventricle. The small cardiac vein (thebesian) drains both atria.

Conduction

Conduction of the heart originates through the sinoatrial node. This sends an impulse to both atria. Next the impulse conducts to the atria ventricle node, which is transmitted to the Purkinje's fibers. This sends an impulse to the ventricles, which contract.

Atrioventricular (AV) node is located in the junction of the right atrium and right ventricle. It merges with the bundle of His. It consists of both parasympathetic and sympathetic innervators.

Sinoatrial (SA) node is located in the junction of the right atrium and superior vena cava. It consists of both parasympathetic and sympathetic innervators and is considered the main pacemaker of the heart.

Purkinje's tissue is located on either side of the intraventricular septum in the right and left branches of the atrioventricular node. It provides special conduction tissue in the ventricles, Purkinje's fibers.

Heart Valves

Aortic Valve

Composed of three semilunar cusps that are located between the left ventricle and aorta. They prevent blood from flowing back into the left ventricle from the aorta. Area to auscultate is the second right intercostal space at the right sternal border (base of heart).

Atrioventricular Valve

A valve in the heart through which blood flows from the atria to the ventricles. This valve prevents backflow of blood into the atria and closes when the ventricular walls contract. The valve located between the left atrium and left ventricle is the mitral valve. The right atrioventricular valve is the tricuspid valve.

Bicuspid or Mitral Valve

Consists of two cusps (bicuspid) and is located between the left atrium and left ventricle. Allows blood to flow from left atrium to left ventricle but closes to prevent backflow of blood into the atrium. Area to auscultate is the fifth left intercostal space at the midclavicular line (apical area).

Pulmonic Valve

Composed of three semilunar cusps that close during each heartbeat to prevent blood from flowing back into the right ventricle from the pulmonary artery. Area to auscultate is the second left intercostal space at the left sternal border.

Tricuspid Valve or Right Atrioventricular Valve

A valve consisting of three main cusps (ventral, dorsal, and medial cusps) and is located between the right atrium and right ventricle of the heart. The tricuspid allows blood flow into ventricles and closes to prevent back flow into the atria. Area to auscultate is fourth left intercostal space along the lower left sternal border.

Heart Tissue

Epicardium

The inner layer of one of the pericardium. One of three layers; it is composed of a single sheet of squamous epithelial.

Endocardium

The lining of the heart chamber composed of small blood vessels and smooth muscles.

Myocardium

The middle layer of the heart composed of thick muscle cells, which form a major portion of the heart wall.

Pericardium

A tough white fibrous sac that surrounds the heart and roots of the great vessels. It consists of the serous pericardium and the fibrous pericardium. It protects the heart and the serous membranes.

Heart Chambers

Left Atrium

Receives oxygenated blood from pulmonary veins. Sends blood into the left ventricle from the atria during diastole.

Left Ventricle

High-pressure circulatory that pumps blood through the aorta and systemic arteries, the capillaries, and back through the veins to the right atrium.

Right Atrium

Sends deoxygenated blood from the superior and inferior vena cava and the coronary sinus into the right ventricle.

Right Ventricle

Low-pressure pump that sends blood from the pulmonary artery to the lungs for oxygenation.

Heart Rate

- Normal: 80 to 100 beats per minute
- Bradycardia: heart rate under 60 beats per minute
- Tachycardia: heart rate above 100 beats per minute
- Maximum heart rate: 220 minus age

Blood Pressure

Systole

The period of cardiac contraction. Correlates with first heart sound when taking blood pressure.

Diastole

The period of cardiac relaxation or filling. Correlates with last heart sound when taking blood pressure.

Normal

Depends on age and will vary.

Age	Systolic	Diastolic
1 month	80	45
6 months	90	60
2 years	80 to 90	55 to 65
4 years	100 to 115	55 to 75
6 years	105 to 125	60 to 80
8 years	105 to 125	665 to 80
10 years	110to 135	65 to 80
12 years	115 to 135	65 to 80
14 years	120 to 140	70 to 85
Adult	110 to 140	60 to 80
Elderly	Slightly higher than adult	Slightly lower than adult

Hypertension

Blood pressure at 140/90 or above must be tested three times to be conclusive.

Hypotension

Abnormally low blood pressure
- Occurs in shock
- Orthostatic hypotension—can occur as a result of patient assuming an upright position; especially common after long periods of bedrest

Heart Sounds

Normal Heart Sounds

1. S1 (lub): atrioventricular valves closing. This is the sound heard when the tricuspid and mitral valves are closing inside the heart.
2. S2 (dub): this is the sound heard when the pulmonic and aortic valves are closing inside the heart.

Abnormal Heart Sounds

1. S3 (ventricular gallop): may be audible immediately following the second heart sound. This would indicate decompensated heart functioning or heart failure if heard in an older person or someone with heart disease. When heard in healthy children, young adults, or athletes, it is considered a physiologically normal sound.
2. S4 (atrial gallop): may be heard immediately preceding the first heart sound and is associated with increased resistance to ventricular filling. Sign of ventricle noncompliance. Often heard in persons with hypertensive heart disease, coronary artery disease, and myocardiopathy.
3. Murmur: turbulent blood flow through a valve. Can be stenosis or prolapsed valve.
4. Pericardial friction rub: inflammation of pericardial sac. High-pitched scratching sound.

Grading System

1	Softest audible murmur
2	Medium audible murmur
3	Loud murmur without thrill
4	Murmur with thrill
5	Loudest murmur that cannot be heard with stethoscope off the chest
6	Audible murmur that can be heard with stethoscope off the chest

EKG Waves

Electrocardiogram (EKG): test that measures the electrical activity of the heart.

Normal

P wave:	Atrial depolarization
QRS complex:	Ventricular depolarization
ST segment:	Pause
T wave:	Ventricular repolarization

Abnormal EKG Readings

- Abnormal P wave could result in an atrial or ventricular arrhythmia.
- QRS wave elevation on an EKG is indicative of possible hypertrophy of the myocardium. QRS wave depression is indicative of possible heart failure or chronic obstructive disorder.
- Abnormally elevated ST segment is indicative of an acute heart attack or a myocardial infarction.
- Abnormal Q wave shows a past history of a possible myocardial infarction. Determining when the infarction occurred is beyond the capabilities of an EKG alone. Clinical follow-up should be performed on the patient to determine the age of the infarct.
- An abnormal or inverted T wave could be indicative of ischemia.

Chapter Eight
Cardiology

Disorders/Diseases

Aneurysm: a bulging of the wall secondary to weakness of the tissue. Aneurysms are usually located in the aorta but may also occur in the peripheral vessels. The arterial aneurysm is usually caused by atherosclerosis, hypertension, or occasionally by trauma, infection, and congenital weakness in the vessel wall. One sign of an arterial aneurysm is a blowing murmur heard on auscultation.

Angina pectoris: a symptom of myocardial ischemia secondary to coronary artery disease. It may be stable, predictable in appearance, occurs after exercise, eating, and exposure to intense cold or emotional stress. Rest, nitrates, or vasodilators typically alleviate this. It may also be unstable, which can occur with activity or rest. This pain is more intense than stable and may last several hours. The pain is typically substernal, epigastrium, and pericardium, with radiation symptoms in the left arm, jaw, or neck. Levels of angina are:
  1+ light or barely noticeable
  2+ moderate or bothersome
  3+ severe and very uncomfortable
  4+ most severe pain ever experienced.

Arrhythmia: a disorder of the electrical activity of the heart causing an absence or irregularity of the heart's normal rhythm.

Atherosclerosis: an arterial disorder that results from an accumulation of plaque, lipids, cholesterol, and cellular debris in the inner layers of the walls of the arteries. The inner layers become progressively thickened, calcification of arterial walls, and a loss of elasticity. This decreases or prevents blood flow through the arteries to the organs. Signs and symptoms may include changes in skin color, headaches, dizziness, intermittent claudication, and changes in peripheral pulses. It may cause a thrombosis and is a major cause of myocardial infarct, angina pectoris, and coronary heart disease.

Atrial septal defect: a congenital heart defect of an abnormal opening between the atria. Atrial septal defect causes an increased flow of oxygenated blood into the right side of the heart. This causes the right heart volume to overload and enlargement of the right atria. The defect is corrected by surgical closure depending on the child's age and severity of the enlargement.

Backward heart failure: venous return to the heart is decreased resulting venous stasis and congestion. Pulmonary edema occurs due to the ventricles not emptying and the blood backing up in the pulmonary veins and lungs.

Cardiac tamponade: accumulation of blood or fluid in the pericardial sac. Signs and symptoms include hypotension, decreased heart sounds, weak or absent peripheral pulses, tachypnea, and pericardial friction rub. It may also be called cardiac compression because of the compression of the heart caused by the accumulation of blood or fluid. Intervention for treatment places the patient on monitored bedrest with aspiration of the blood or fluid. Surgical intervention if necessary to repair the bleeding vessel or vessels.

Congestive heart failure: an impaired cardiac pumping that results in edema and systemic congestion. Left heart failure results from an inability of the left ventricles to pump blood into the systemic circulation. This results in elevated end diastolic left ventricular pressure and pulmonary congestion, fatigue, central cyanosis, cardiac asthma, tachycardia, and pulmonary edema. Hypertension, aortic valve disease, or cardiac failure may cause left heart failure. Right heart failure results in elevated end diastolic right ventricular pressure. This causes systemic congestion, fatigue, cyanosis of the capillary stasis, pleural effusion, enlarged liver, and pitting edema. Mitral stenosis, ineffective endocarditis, and tricuspid valvular disease may cause right heart failure.

Forward heart failure: left ventricle failure results in a greatly reduced cardiac output. This may be caused by loss of contractility of the ventricle or after myocardial infarction.

Heart failure: a condition that results in the heart not being able to pump enough blood to meet the metabolic needs of the body. There are five types of heart failure as follows:

High-output heart failure: cardiac heart failure from an increased amount of circulation. This may be caused by anemia or large arteriovenous fistula.

Low-output heart failure: the heart cannot maintain adequate circulation due to a decreased venous return. This may be caused by a hemorrhage.

Myocardial infarction: also called heart attack; it results in necrosis of a portion of the cardiac muscle. The necrosis or death of the heart muscle tissue is caused by obstruction in the coronary artery. This may be caused by a spasm, thrombus, atherosclerotic heart disease, embolism, and drug overdoses. The myocardial infarction sites may include the right coronary artery, causing an inferior myocardial infarction; circumflex artery, causing a lateral myocardial infarction; and the left descending artery, causing an anterior myocardial infarction. Signs and symptoms include chest pain, sense of heaviness in the chest, nausea, vomiting, sweating, hypotension, weakness, shortness of breath, light headness, and chest pain radiating to the left arm and neck. Myocardial enzymes are released into the blood as a result of necrosis. Blood enzyme and an electrocardiograph may be utilized to assist with patent diagnosis.

Patent ductus arteriosus: a congenital heart defect resulting in an abnormal opening between the pulmonary artery and aorta. The patent duct, located between the descending aorta and pulmonary artery, is bifurcate and does not close after birth. This allows left to right blood flow from the aorta to the pulmonary artery, causing increased workload on the left side of the heart. Surgery is utilized to correct the defect if there is no spontaneous closing and the child is old enough to tolerate the procedure.

Tetralogy of Fallot: a congenital heart defect that results in four specific defects causing a mixing of oxygenated and unoxygenated blood. The four defects are as follows: ventricular septal defect, malpositioning of the aorta, pulmonary stenosis, right ventricular hypertrophy. Surgery is utilized to correct the defect, optimally after the child is 1 year old; and supportive measures are utilized early on to assist the child with comfort and function.

Transposition of the great arteries: a congenital heart defect resulting in the great arteries being reversed. The aorta leaves the right ventricle and pulmonary artery leaves the left ventricle. This prevents communication between the systemic and pulmonary circulation. Surgery is utilized to correct the defect, optimally after the child is at least 6 months of age; and supportive measures are utilized early on to assist the child with comfort and function.

Ventricular septal defect: a congenital heart defect resulting in an opening in the ventricular septum. This allows mixing of the left ventricle's oxygenated blood with the right ventricle's unoxygenated blood. The defect is corrected by surgical closure unless it is small and could close spontaneously.

Cardiac Diagnostic Test

Cardiac catheterization: the coronary arteries are injected with a contrast material for visualization through a cinefluoroscopy or x-ray. This is utilized to determine cardiac output, measure pulmonary artery and blood gas pressure, abnormal wall movements, ventricular function, and anatomy of the heart.

Echocardiography: the reflections of ultrasound waves from the cardiac surfaces are analyzed. This is utilized to determine left ventricular systolic functioning, observe chambers, evaluate movement of valves, and evaluate structure and function of cardiac walls. This can assist in identifying tumors or pericardial effusion.

Electrocardiogram: 12 surface electrodes are placed on the patient to record the electrical activity of the patient's heart. The electrodes will provide feedback on cardiac rhythm, rate, conduction, and myocardial infarctions or ischemia.

Exercise stress test: an exercise test preformed typically on a stationary bike or treadmill where the physician can monitor the patient's response to a variety of exercise levels. Typically, heart rate, blood pressure, respiratory rate, patient's perceived level of exertion/workload, and electrocardiogram are monitored to provide feedback to how the patient's cardiovascular system responds under stress.

Holter monitoring: electrocardiograph reading with an ambulatory EKG unit to monitor patient for typically 24 hours. This monitors the patient while performing normal activities. Utilized to monitor the effects of medication, activities of daily living, ambulation, pacemaker functions, and evaluation of patient's symptoms with patient's daily activities.

Phonocardiography: an electroacoustic device that will produce and record heart sounds. A microphone is placed over the base of the heart and on the chest over the apex of the heart. This records aortic and pulmonary components of the heart sounds. This information is utilized to confirm auscultatory findings.

Radionuclide angiocardiography: red blood cells marked with radionuclide are injected into the blood. They are then monitored to determine ventricular wall motion, ejection fraction, congenital defects, and abnormal blood flow.

Technetium 99m scanning: the patient's blood is injected with technetium 99m, a radionuclide, which is taken up by the myocardial tissue. This is also called hot spot imaging and is utilized to evaluate and located myocardial infarctions.

Thallium 201 myocardial perfusion imaging: thallium 201 is injected into the blood at the patient's peak exercise level. This is also called cold spot imaging and is utilized to identify ischemia myocardium, infarcted myocardium, and diagnosis coronary artery disease.

Treatment Options

Angioplasty

Also called percutaneous transluminal coronary angioplasty, it is a nonsurgical technique for coronary artery disease (atherosclerosis). A balloon tipped catheter is inserted and inflated under the radiographic or ultrasonic visual field. The balloon is inflated and deflated until it is confirmed that there is arterial dilation and reduces pressure in the artery. The balloon-tip catheter is then removed from the patient and the artery is left unoccluded. The angioplasty also helps alleviate anginal pain. This procedure's advantage over bypass surgery is that the patient does not have to undergo open chest surgery, thereby eliminating the risks associated with surgery and having a shorter recovery period.

Coronary Artery Bypass Graft (CABG)

An open-heart surgical technique utilized to bypass clogged, blocked, and narrowing vessels. The saphenous vein, from the patient's leg, is used as a graft to route blood around the blockage to an alternative route to the heart. Another option for the graft is to use the internal mammary artery. It is possible for the patient to have double, triple, and quadruple bypass surgery. This is utilized to relieve anginal pain and improve blood flow to the heart muscle.

Coronary Stents

A coronary stent may be utilized on a severely occluded or blocked coronary artery.

The surgical procedure involves placing a stent in the occluded artery to keep the artery open and maintain a normal blood flow. The stent allows the blood to flow to the heart muscle. A balloon expandablestent is placed in the artery to keep it open; the balloon can be inflated to open the artery up to normal blood flow and is left inside the patient. An advantage to the stent over angioplasty and coronary artery bypass graft is that the stents require less repeat surgeries. Approximately 30% of patients receiving angioplasty and coronary artery bypass grafts have repeated surgery due to renarrowing of the arteries within 3 years.

Transplantation

- Patients are accepted as heart transplantation candidates because they cannot survive without the transplantation.
- Patients may also be considered candidates if they have an ejection fraction of less then 20%.
- Absolute contraindications include uncontrolled malignancy or infections.
- Other possible contraindications are individual and decided by each facility.
- Homologous transplants are from another human.
- Orthotopic homologous transplantation refers to the grafting of the donor heart into the normal heart site.
- Heterotopic homologous transplantation refers to when the patient's heart remains intact and the donor's heart is placed parallel.
- Post-transplantation concerns include infections and rejection.
- Physical therapy starts in the coronary care unit (CCU).

Ventricular Assistive Device

- A mechanical device also called a left ventricular assistive device (LAVD).
- This device is being developed to help patient's stay alive while awaiting heart surgery.
- The device provides circulatory support by pumping blood through the body.

Medication Therapy*

A wide variety of medications may be utilized in treatment of cardiac disease and disorders. Medications may be used to alleviate symptoms (eg, nitroglycerin to decrease angina pain). Listed below are samples of pharmacology agents that are used in cardiac treatments:

1. **Antiarrhythmics**
   - Used to alleviate, prevent, or correct a cardiac arrhymia
   - Alters conductivity
   - Prolongs the refractory period
   - Improves cardiac output
   - Goal is to have diastolic at 90 or lower
   - Quinidine, disopyramide, and procainamide

---

*Commonly known drug names are listed in this section. Please note that some are generic or chemical names and some are brand names.

2. Anticoagulants
- Used to prevent blood clot formation
- Coumadin, asprin, and platelet inhibitors

3. Antihypertensives
- Reduces high blood pressure
- Reduces myocardial oxygen demands
- Decreases myocardial force and rate of contraction
- Diazoxide, guanethidine, and propranolol

4. Beta Adrenergic Blocking Agents
- Reduces blood pressure
- Decreases rate and force of heart contractions
- Blocks sympathetic conduction at B-receptors
- Also utilized for angina, arrhythmias, and hypertension
- Acebutolol, metoprolol, Lopressor, Inderal, and propranolol

5. Calcium Channel Blocking Agents
- Inhibits the flow of calcium ions across the membranes of smooth muscle cells
- Lowers heart rate and blood pressure
- Helps to control chest pain and arrhythmias
- Relaxes smooth muscle tone
- Diltiazem (Cardizem), nifedipine (Procardia), and verapamil

6. Digitalis
- Decreases heart rate
- Increases myocardial contractions
- Slowing down of A-V nodal conductors
- More regular apical heart rate
- Used to inhibit atrial flutter, congestive heart failure, congenital heart block, and myocarditis
- Dosage must be monitored for toxicity
- Digoxin is used for congestive heart failure patients

7. Diuretics
- Reduces the volume of extracellular fluid
- Controls fluid retention
- Reduces myocardial workload
- Used for hypertension, congestive heart failure, and edema
- Most common drug is Lasix; Diuril and Aldactone are also used

8. **Lipid-Lowering Drugs**
   - Decreases serum lipid levels
   - Interferes with metabolism of blood fats
   - Lowers cholesterol
   - Used to assist in prevention of atherosclerosis
   - Colestrid, Lopid, Mevocor, and Zocor

9. **Nitrates**
   - Dilates coronary arteries
   - Reduces angina pain
   - Improves coronary blood flow
   - Most common is nitroglycerin
   - Isodril, Iso-bid, and isosorbide dinitrate

10. **Vasodilators**
   - Dilates the peripheral blood vessels
   - Used in combination with diuretics
   - Nitroglycerin and isosorbide dinitrate

Cardiac Rehabilitation

Risk Factors Associated With Heart Disease

- Smoking
- Hypertension
- Elevated cholesterol levels
- Family history
- Sedentary lifestyle
- Diabetes
- Age
- Male gender

Overall Treatment for Cardiac Disease

- Diet
- Medication
- Exercise
- Behavioral changes

Note: A multiphasic approach to risk factor reduction is key. No single element alone is an effective treatment.

Cardiac Response to Exercise

Normal Response

1. Under normal conditions the cardiac output and heart rate will increase in a linear relationship with the increase in work load and oxygen consumption demand.

2. Maximum heart rate will decrease with age (220 minus age = maximum heart rate).

3. Blood pressure: systolic will rise but diastolic will remain level or slightly increase.

Abnormal Response

1. On EKG, the ST segment will depress or elevate, denoting heart injury.

2. Blood pressure:
   • Systolic: will remain level during exercise or remain high after exercise
   • Diastolic: will increase above 20 mmHg or decrease after exercise

3. Angina symptoms during exercise

4. Abnormal heart rate—bradycardia or tachycardia
   *Note: **Stop** exercising the patient if any of the above occur during exercise. Continue to monitor pulse and blood pressure while calling for assistance.*

Possible Benefits of a Cardiac Rehabilitation Program

- Decreases serum lipid level
- Improves maximum oxygen consumption
- Increases HDL levels
- May decrease high blood pressure
- Improves activity/exercise tolerance
- Improves or relieves angina
- Improves aerobic capacity
- Decreases depression following myocardial infarction
- Decreases heart rate at rest
- Improves heart rate recovery after exercise
- Improves respiratory capacity during exercise
- Increases stoke volume
- Assists in weight reduction

Energy Costs of Selected Activites—MET Levels

Metabolic equivalents (METS) are used to compare the energy costs of various activities to rest.

Level	Activities
1 ½ to 2 METS	Sitting, self-feeding, reading, active assistive exercise to extremities in supine or sitting, standing, walking (1 mph), desk work
2 to 3 METS	Typing, level walking (2 mph), level bicycling (5 mph), light woodworking, playing an instrument, active exercise standing or light mat activities, light weights (2 to 3 pounds) may be used, lawn mowing with a riding mower
3 to 4 METS	Cleaning windows, walking (3 mph), cycling (6 mph), archery, golf (pulling the golf bag cart), fishing, slow stair-climbing, balance and mat activities with mild resistance
4 to 5 METS	House painting, walking to 3.5 mph, cycling (8 mph), raking leaves, light dancing, resistance exercise sitting to 10 to 15 pounds maximum
5 to 6 METS	Shoveling light soil, walking (4 mph), horseback riding, ice skating, stairs/step aerobics to tolerance, hand lawn mowing
6 to 7 METS	Shoveling 10 pounds, cycling (11 mph), light snow shoveling, light downhill skiing, walking (5 mph)
7 to 10 METS	Jogging to rapid running, basketball, heavy shoveling, vigorous skiing, rapid cycling up and down hills, cycling (13 mph), horseback riding/galloping, walking (5.5 mph)
11 to 12 METS	Backpacking, climbing hills, handball, racquetball, jumping rope 120 to 140 skips/minute, running 5-minute mile
13 to 14 METS	Running 7-minute mile, cross-country skiing vigorously, shoveling wet snow

Cardiac Rehabilitation Program

Contraindications for Cardiac Rehabilitation Program Participation

- Unstable angina
- Fever
- Thrombophlebitis
- Uncontrolled diabetes
- Acute illness
- Uncontrolled dysrhythmias
- Uncontrolled tachycardia
- Recent embolism
- Third-degree heart block
- Symptomatic congestive heart failure
- Resting systolic blood pressure over 200 mmHg
- Resting diastolic blood pressure over 100 mmHg

Borg 10-Grade Scale for Perceived Exertion

0	Nothing
0.5	Very, very weak
1.0	Very weak
1.5	Weak (light)
3.0	Moderate
4.0	Somewhat strong
5.0	Strong (heavy)
6.0	
7.0	Very strong
8.0	
9.0	
10.0	Very, very strong (almost maximum)

Exercise Prescription

1. Intensity
- Cardiac patient should have an exercise stress test prior.
- The cardiac patient should initially start at a low-level intensity.
- Age adjusted heart rate for maximum is 220 minus the patient's age. This can then be multiplied by 65% to 95% to determine work-load level.
- 50% to 85% of maximum oxygen consumption.

2. Duration
- Fifteen to 60 minutes of scheduled exercise period.

3. Frequency
- Three to 5 days per week with no more than 2 days of rest between sessions.

Phase I—Inpatient Cardiac Rehabilitation

- Phase I is the beginning protocol for the patient's cardiac rehabilitation programs. This begins as an inpatient in the coronary care unit. Phase I is the acute phase.
- It may include some of the following activity levels:
  1. Monitored ambulation, which typically uses Holter monitoring and involves monitoring the patient's heart and blood pressure while the patient is ambulating with the physical therapist or cardiac nurse.
  2. Passive range of motion (ROM), ankle pumps and breathing exercises progressing to active ROM supine, active ROM sitting, walking 50 to 75 feet.
  3. Phase I may also include low-level exercise testing.
  4. ADL training for bathroom procedures is typical.
  5. Ward activities start and progress; bedside commode, feeding, and partial self care; sitting in chair 15 minutes to 30 minutes; showers; dressing; bathroom privilege; and exercise testing.
  6. Calisthenics progressing from 1.0 to 4.0 METS.
  7. Education on pulse monitoring, activity diary, blood pressure, nutrition, home exercise program, and exercise prescriptions.
- Discharged after a submaximal or low-level treadmill test.

Phase II—Outpatient Cardiac Rehabilitation

- Phase II is considered an outpatient cardiac rehabilitation program. This is conducted after the patient is discharged from phase I and enters outpatient cardiac rehabilitation. Phase II is the subacute phase.
- Phase II program includes an increase in the patient's exercise program, again with continued monitoring. Phase II also includes continued patient education, typically regarding risk factors, diets, stress, and medication.

- Phase II includes more aggressive stress testing for the patient.
- Phase II is typically an 8 to 12 week program. Payers (insurance companies) typically cover 36 sessions, which are usually scheduled three times a week for 12 weeks.
- Duration of exercise is usually 30 to 60 minutes per session.
- It begins with the completion of a low-level treadmill test and ends with the maximal treadmill test. MET functional level at exit is typically nine.
- Phase II may include some of the following activities:
  1. Group support program
  2. Walking
  3. Treadmill
  4. Ergometer
  5. Circuit training
  6. Risk factor modification
  7. Teach energy conservation techniques
  8. Patients should now be independent in self monitoring or vital signs

Phase III—Community Exercise Program

- Phase III is typically referred to as a maintenance program. It is the process of ongoing exercise performed by the patient under supervised conditions of a self-regulated exercise program.
- Phase III is a high-level exercise conditioning phase. Patients exercise at 65% to 85% of their maximum heart rate, which is obtained from their treadmill test.
- Duration is typically 45 to 60 minutes per session.
- Frequency is a minimum of three times a week and may be daily.
- Discharge is typically 6 to 12 months.
- Supervision during the exercise session is still encouraged.
- Insurance does not typically cover the maintenance program and patient's may exercise at a community center, private club, or a hospital-based program if available.

Phase IV—Ongoing for Life

- Phase IV is promoting a life-long commitment to cardiac care, including exercise, diet, and behavior modification.

Goals of the Cardiac Rehabilitation Program

Phase I

Some examples include the following:
- Assessment of the patient's response to activities of daily living and self care.
- Determining the patient's response to monitored ambulation activities.
- Assisting the patient in identifying risk factors and methods to reduce them.
- Educating the family.
- Identifying diet and medication assessment.
- Patient should be able to pass a mild stress test.

All these areas may be assessed during phase I and appropriate goals set up for the patient. For example, one specific goal under education might be for the patient to independently list the risk factors associated with his or her evaluation and identify what steps he or she can take to modify those risks.

Phase II

Some examples of goals include the following:
- Determining the patient's response to exercise in a safe manner.
- Evaluating the home environment for the patient's transition from an inpatient to outpatient basis.
- Assessing whether response to exercise is appropriate.
- Monitoring the patient's social and emotional response to the program.
- Patient should be able to pass a maximal stress test.

Phase III

Some examples of maintenance goals include the following:
- Patient should be able to exercise independently in a safe manner.
- The patient should be educated in independent management of risk factors, medication, diet, and stress.
- Patient should be able to independently perform activities of daily living in a safe manner.

Chapter Nine

Pulmonary Anatomy & Physiology

Lung Structure

The lungs are divided into a right lung, which contains three lobes, and a left lung, which contains two lobes. The right lung consists of 10 segments. The left lung consists of eight segments. The pleura is a delicate membrane enclosing the lung. The pleura is divided into the visceral pleura, which covers the lungs, and the parietal pleura, which lines the chest wall and covers the diaphragm. The pleural cavity is the space within the thorax that contains the lungs. The pleural space is the potential space between the visceral and parietal layers of the pleura. It contains a small amount of fluid that acts as a lubricant.

Upper and Lower Airways

The upper airway entry point into the respiratory system is the nose or mouth. The pharynx serves as a passageway for the respiratory and digestive tracts. The pharynx is composed of muscle, is lined with a mucous membrane, and contains the opening of the larynx. The larynx is the air passage that connects the pharynx with the trachea. The trachea conveys air to the lungs. The trachea starts the lower airways. At the fifth thoracic vertebra, the trachea divides into two bronchi: primary and secondary. The bronchiole extends from the bronchi into the lobes of the lung. The terminal branches allow passively inspired air from the bronchi to the respiratory bronchioles. The respiratory bronchioles allow the exchange of air and waste gases between the alveolar ducts and the terminal bronchioles.

Muscles of Inspiration

Inspiratory muscles act to draw air into the lungs to exchange oxygen for carbon dioxide. The major muscle of inspiration is the diaphragm.

Primary

- Diaphragm phrenic innervation (C3, C4, C5)
- Levatores costarum
- External intercostal
- Internal intercostal

Accessory

- Scaleni
- Sternocleidomastoid
- Trapezius
- Serratus anterior—posterior superior
- Pectoralis major
- Pectoralis minor
- Latissimus dorsi
- Thoracic spine extensors
- Subclavius

Muscles of Expiration

Expiration is the moving of air out of the lungs, or exhalation. Expiration is a result of passive relaxation of inspiratory muscles and elastic recoil of lungs.

Primary

- Internal oblique
- External oblique
- Rectus abdominis
- Transverse abdominis
- Internal intercostal—posterior
- Transverse thoracic

Accessory

- Latissimus dorsi
- Serratus anterior—posterior inferior
- Iliocostalis lumborum
- Quadratus lumborum

Breathing Sounds

Normal

- **Bronchial:** inspiration shorter than expiration. Short pause between inspiration and expiration. Loud and high pitched.

- **Bronchovesicular:** inspiration equals expiration in duration, with no pause between. Lower intensity than bronchial. Medium pitched.

- **Tracheal:** inspiration and expiration are equal in duration. Short pause between inspiration and expiration. Loud and high pitched.

- **Vesicular:** longer inspiration and shorter expiration with no pause between. Relatively faint and low pitched.

Abnormal

- **Bronchophony:** an increase in intensity and clarity of vocal resonance. This may result in an increase in lung tissue density (eg, pneumonia).

- **Crackles:** result of secretions, as in pneumonia or early tuberculosis. Characterized by popping or bubbling sounds.

- **Egophony:** a change in voice sound when a patient is asked to make an "e" sound and it sounds like an "a" over the peripheral chest wall. May be caused by pleural effusion.

- **Friction rub:** a dry, grating sound similar to footsteps on packed snow. Caused by rubbing of pleural surfaces against one another.

- **Pectoriloquy:** abnormal transmission of whispered syllables that cannot be heard clearly.

- **Rhonchi:** airways obstructed by thick secretions, muscular spasm, neoplasm, or external pressure causing a continuous rumbling sound.

- **Wheeze:** a high-pitched musical quality, caused by airway obstruction. Airways may be narrowed by inflammation of secretions or bronchospasm.

Division of Left and Right Lungs

Left Lung (Eight Segments)

Left Upper Lobe	Left Lower Lobe
ap = apical—posterior	s = superior
an = anterior	ab = anterior medial basal
sl = superior lingula	lb = lateral basal
il = inferior lingula	pb = posterior basal

Right Lung (10 Segments)

Right Upper Lobe	Right Middle Lobe	Right Lower Lobe
ap = apical	l = lateral	s = superior
an = anterior basal	m = medial	ab = anterior
p = posterior		lb = lateral basal
		pb = posterior basal
		mb = medial basal

Evaluation of Sputum

Sputum is described in terms of quantity, viscosity, color, and odor. The color will assist in determining the condition that the patient is experiencing.

- Red: blood
- Pink: pulmonary edema
- Yellow: infection starting to clear
- Green: acute infection
- Gray: abscess
- Rust: pneumonia
- White or clear: may equal chronic cough or cystic fibrosis or chronic bronchitis
- Thick tenacious sputum: asthmatic bronchitis

Chapter Ten

Pulmonary Diseases & Disorders

Pulmonary Diseases/Disorders

Asthma

- Increased sensitivity of trachea and bronchi to irritants
- Spasms of smooth bronchi muscle
- Narrowing of airway
- Inflammation and production of mucus
- Increased respiratory rate
- Chest wall movements normal or symmetrically decreased
- Dry, irritating, or wheezing cough
- Symptoms may include anxiety, bronchial spasm

Adult Respiratory Distress Syndrome

- Respiratory syndrome characterized by hypoxemia and respiratory deficiency
- May be caused by aspiration of a foreign object, oxygen toxicity, trauma, pneumonia, respiratory infections, and multiple blood transfusions
- Patient may demonstrate tachypnea, hypoxemia, breathlessness, and decreased lung compliance
- Other names for this include acute respiratory distress syndrome, shock lung, wet lung, pump lung, and congestive atelectasis

Atelectasis

- Collapsed or airless alveolar unit
- Prevents the respiratory exchange of oxygen and carbon dioxide

- May be caused by internal bronchial obstruction, postoperative pain, external bronchial compression, narcotic overdose, rib fracture, and neurological trauma
- Patient may demonstrate decreased breathing sounds, tachycardia, increased temperature, and dyspnea

Bronchiectasis

- Abnormal condition of the bronchial tree
- Chest wall movement may be reduced over effected side
- Increased vocal sounds
- Sputum possibly foul smelling and hemoptysis may occur
- Characterized by irreversible dilatation and destruction of the bronchial walls
- Symptoms include a constant cough with sputum, chronic sinusitis, clubbing of fingers
- Treatment includes postural drainage, antibiotics

Bronchogenic Carcinoma

- A malignant lung tumor that originates in the bronchi
- May cause coughing, fatigue, chest tightness, aching joints
- Surgery is the most effective treatment; however, approximately 50% of cases are advanced and inoperable
- Treatment can include radiotherapy and chemotherapy

Bronchopulmonary Dysplasia

- Obstructive pulmonary disease
- The lungs have abnormal development and pulmonary immaturity
- Seen in premature infants
- Symptoms may include decreased breath sounds, increased bronchial secretions, crackles/wheezing, and hyperinflation

Chronic Bronchitis

- Distinguished by excessive secretion of mucus in the bronchi, including a productive cough for at least 3 consecutive months
- Other symptoms may include chest infections, cyanosis, hypoxemia and hypercapnia, wheezing and rhonchi
- Chest wall movement normal or symmetrically decreased

- Normal vocal sounds
- Productive cough with sputum with infection
- Treatment includes cessation of cigarette smoking, postural drain

Cystic Fibrosis

- Genetically determined systemic disease of the exocrine glands
- Increased secretions with rales and wheezing
- Overproduction of mucus
- Congenital disease
  Chest walls movement normal or reduced
- Vocal sounds may have egophony
- Cough is productive and sputum may have hemoptysis

Emphysema

- Lung tissue loses its elasticity
- Lungs remain overinflated; diaphragm flattens and is then less effective
- Destruction of alveolar walls allows airways to collapse
- Barrel chest
- Pink puffers
- Chest wall movement normal or symmetrically reduced
- Vesicular breath sounds
- Patient's cough and sputum variable

Hemothorax

- Blood and fluid in the pleural cavity between the parietal and visceral pleura
- Usually a result of trauma
- Emergency care necessary, as shock may occur from hemorrhage, pain, and respiratory failure
- Symptoms may include chest pain, respiratory distress, signs of blood loss, and decreased breath sounds

Hyaline Membrane Disease

- Respiratory distress syndrome of the newborn (RDS)—acute lung disease
- Characterized by airless alveoli, inelastic lungs, more than 60 res-

piration per minute, nasal flaring, intercostal and subcostal retractions, grunting on expiration and peripheral edema
- Most often in premature babies
- Treatment includes measures to correct shock, acidosis, and hypoxemia and use of continuous positive airway pressure especially developed for infants

Lung Contusion

- Blood and edema within the alveoli and interstitial space
- The injury does not break the skin
- Caused by trauma or a blow to the lung area
- Symptoms may include swelling, pain, decreased breath sounds, and cyanosis

Peripheral Airway Disease

- Inflammation of distal conducting airways
- Associated with smokers and obesity
- Decrease in forced expiratory flow (FEF) 25 to 75%

Pneumonia

- Chest wall movement reduced on effected side
- Breath sounds are vesicular or bronchial
- Vocal sounds are egophony, or whispering pectoriloquy
  - **Aspiration pneumonia** is an inflammatory condition of the lungs and bronchi. It is caused by inhalation of foreign matter or vomitus containing acid gastric contents.
  - **Bacterial pneumonia** is a bacteria infection in the interalveolar. The most common type is streptococcal. Symptoms may include fever, cough, shaking chills, crackle sound, and decreased breath sounds.
  - **Viral pneumonia** is a pulmonary infection caused by a virus.

Pneumothorax

- A collection of air or gas in the pleural space, which causes the lung to collapse
- May be the result of an open chest wound that permits entrance of air

- Onset is a sudden, sharp chest pain followed by difficult rapid breaths
- Cessation of normal chest wall movements on effected side
- Vocal sounds decreased
- A dry cough
- Symptoms may include local or referred pain, chest pain, cyanosis
- Treatment includes being placed in bed in Fowler's position, oxygen unless contraindicated, and air aspirated from the pleural space. Intermittent positive pressure breathing may be administered. Educate the patient on passive exercise, how to turn, cough, and breathe deeply

Pulmonary Edema

- Excessive fluid from the pulmonary vascular system into the interstitial space
- Chest wall movement is normal or symmetrically reduced
- Vocal sounds are normal
- Cough may include frothy white or pink sputum
- Symptoms may include rales, crackles, dyspnea, and tachypnea

Pulmonary Effusion

- Excessive fluid between the visceral and parietal pleura
- Reduced or absent chest wall movement on the effected side
- Breath sounds are decreased or absent; high-pitched bronchial may be present
- Vocal sounds are reduced or absent
- May have pleural rub
- Cough is absent or nonproductive
- Symptoms may include pain and/or fever

Pulmonary Embolism

- A thrombus that becomes embolic and is lodged in the pulmonary circulation
- Chest wall movement is reduced on the effected side
- Breath sounds may be reduced
- Vocal sounds are normal
- Symptoms may include wheezing, pleural friction rub, rales, dry hacking cough with hemoptysis, and possible pleuritic pain

Rib Fracture

- A break in the bone of thoracic skeleton
- May be caused by a blow, crushing injury, or violent coughing
- Most common rib fracture occurs at the fourth to eighth ribs
- Breathing is rapid and shallow
- Site of break is tender to the touch
- Symptoms may include decreased or absent breath sounds, rales and rhonchi, crackling of bone fragments rubbing together
- Confirmation by chest x-ray

Tuberculosis (TB)

- Chronic granulomatous infection caused by an acid-fast bacillus
- Transmitted by inhalation or ingestion of infected droplets
- Listlessness, vague chest pain, pleurisy, fever, and weight loss
- Hospitalization for the first weeks of treatment with a combination of drugs, rest and good nutrition

Respiratory Diseases

Obstructive Versus	Restrictive
Something interferes with the normal airflow	Reduction of actual lung volume
Increased secretions	Structural deformity
Spasms	Chest wall stiffness
Inflammation	Loss of lung tissue
May be reversible	Difficult to treat
Examples: asthma, cystic fibrosis, emphysema, bronchitis, pulmonary edema	Examples: scoliosis, pectus excavatum, burns, pneumothorax, collagen diseases, neuromuscular diseases

Clinical Presentation in COPD (Chronic Bronchitis and Emphysema)

Blue Bloater	Versus	Pink Puffer
Chronic productive cough		Little sputum, shortness of breath
Obese, edematous, cyanotic		Thin, nonedematous, pink
Right side congestive heart failure		Typically no congestive heart failure
Inflammatory cells in submucosa, edema		Destruction of airways
Hypertrophy of bronchial, smooth muscles		

Pulmonary Function Test

Obstructive Versus Restrictive

Test	Obstructive	Restrictive
Total lung capacity	Increases	Decreases
PCO_2	Increases	Decreases
FEV1	Sharply decreases	Normal
Functional residual capacity	Increases	Decreases
Residual volume	Increases	Decreases
Vital capacity	Decreases	Decreases
Vital capacity as a percent of predicted value	Normal > 80%	
	Mild obstructive 80%	
	Mild restrictive 60 to 80%	
	Severe obstructive < 80%	
	Severe restrictive < 50%	
FEV1/FVC ratio	Normal > 75%	
	Mild obstructive 60 to 75%	
	Moderate obstructive 40 to 60%	
	Severe obstructive < 40%	
	Restrictive—normal	

Pulmonary Diagnostic Testing

Arterial Blood Gas

The oxygen and carbon dioxide in arterial blood is measured by various methods to assess the adequacy of ventilation and oxygenation, as well as the acid base status. The normal pH of arterial blood is 7.4.

Auscultation

Listening to lung sounds, typically through a stethoscope. The examiner listens for the frequency, duration, intensity, and quality of sounds. The areas evaluated include tracheal, bronchial, bronchovesicular, and vesicular.

Bronchoscopy

The visual examination of the tracheobronchial tree utilizing a standard rigid, tubular metal bronchoscope or a narrower, flexible fiberoptic bronchoscope. The patient should have fasted and typically is sedated before the examination.

Fluoroscopy

A technique in radiology for visually examining a part of the body or the function of an organ using a fluoroscope. This technique delivers immediate serial images.

Graded Exercise Test

This is a test designed to evaluate a patient's cardiopulmonary response to progressively increasing exercise. The patient's arterial blood gases and/or pulse oximetry are evaluated throughout testing. Pulmonary function testing is performed before and after the graded exercise test.

Exercise termination criteria: the test should be stopped upon any of the following indications:
- Maximal shortness of breath
- Total fatigue
- Leg pain
- Symptoms of fatigue

- Reaching ventilatory maximum
- Insufficient cardiac output
- Cardiac ischemia
- Cardiac dysrhythmias
- Increase in diastolic blood pressure of 20 mmHg
- Decrease in blood pressure with increased workloads
- Fall in Pao_2 of >20 mmHg or a Pao_2 <55 mmHg
- Rise in $Paco_2$ of >10 mmHg or a $Paco_2$ >65 mmHg

Percussion

An evaluation technique in which the therapist will strike the distal end of the middle finger of one hand over the middle finger of the other hand. The hand is placed firmly over the chest wall of the patient. The examiner evaluates the percussion sounds to determine if they are flat, dull, normal, or hyper-resonant.

Pulmonary Function Test

A series of tests that measure the lung capacity, volumes, and flow rates. These tests determine the capacity of the lungs to exchange oxygen and carbon dioxide. The tests performed can include tidal volume, inspiratory reserve volume, expiratory reserve volume, residual volume, and vital capacity.

Spirometer

A laboratory evaluation of the air capacity of the lungs through use of the spirometer. The spirometer measures and records the volume of air inhaled and exhaled. The information is recorded on a chart called a spirometric.

Sputum Studies

A patient's sputum is evaluated to determine the presence of cancer cells, bacteria, and to identify bacteria sensitivity to antibiotic treatments. A gram study can be preformed to identify the category of bacteria (gram positive or negative) and its appearance. The sputum can be cultured for identification and sensitivity to treatment with antibiotics. Cytology reports and evaluation can identify the presence of cancer cells in the sputum.

Color evaluation: the color will assist in determining the condition of the patient.

- Red = blood
- Pink = pulmonary edema
- Yellow = infection starting to clear
- Green = acute infection
- Gray = abscess
- Rust = pneumonia
- Thick tenacious sputum = asthmatic bronchitis

Ventilation Perfusion (V/Q) Scan

Matches the ventilation pattern of the lung to the perfusion pattern. This is done to identify the presence of pulmonary emboli.

X-ray (Roentgen Ray)

Electromagnetic radiation of shorter wavelength than visible light. It is produced when electrons traveling at high speed strike certain materials. It can be used to investigate the integrity of structures, to therapeutically destroy dead tissue, and to make photographic images for diagnostic purposes.

Pulmonary Pharmacology

Antibiotics

Antimicrobial agents derived from cultures of a microorganism or produced semisynthetically and used to treat infections by destroying or interfering with the development of a living organism.

- Erythromycin
- Penicillin
- Tetracycline

Antihistamines

- Azatadine
- Brompheniramine
- Dimenhydrinate
- Diphenhydramine
- Loratadine
- Phenindamine

Bronchodilators

- Epinephrine
- Isoproterenol
- Metaproterenol
- Terbutaline
- Salbutamol
- Theophylline
- Albuterol
- Procaterol

Corticosteroids

- Glucocorticoids—prednisone
- Mineral corticoids—aldosterones
- Dexamethasone
- Prednisolone
- Triamcinolone

Mucokinetics

- Bland aerosol
- Acetylcysteine—reduces viscosity of secretions

Oxygen

- Odorless, tasteless, colorless transparent gas that is slightly heavier than air.
  1. Low-flow oxygen therapy: provides only part of the patient's required minute volume.
  2. High-flow oxygen therapy: provides all of the gas the patient needs.

Lung Volumes

- **Dead air space:** area in which no gas exchange takes place.

- **Residual volume (RV):** amount of gas left over after maximum expiration, which helps prevent the lungs from collapsing.

- **Tidal volume (TV):** amount of gas inspired and expired at rest.

- **Forced expiratory volume (FEV):** amount of air that can be forcibly expelled after maximum inspiration.

- **Total lung capacity (TLC):** amount of gas in the respiratory system after a maximal inspiration.

- **Vital capacity (VC):** maximum volume of air forcibly expired after a maximal inspiration.

- **Inspiratory capacity (IC):** maximum volume of air inspired from resting level of expiratory air.

- **Functional residual capacity (FRC):** volume of gas in lungs after normal expiration.

- **Inspiratory reserve volume (IRV):** maximum volume inspired after normal inspiration.

- **Expiratory reserve volume (ERV):** maximum volume expired after normal expiration.

Pulmonary Classes of Impairment

Class 1—0% Impairment

1. Roentgenographic appearance is usually normal but may show healed or inactive disease
2. Dyspnea may occur but is consistent with the activity
3. FEV and FVC (forced vital capacity) tests are not less then 85% of predicted value
4. Arterial oxygen saturation is not applicable

Class 2—20% to 30% Impairment

1. Roentgenographic appearance may be either normal or abnormal
2. Dyspnea does not occur at rest and during the performance of usual activities of daily living. Patients comparable to person of same age and body build on level surfaces but not unleveled
3. FEV and FVC tests are 70 to 85% predicted value
4. Arterial saturation is not applicable

Class 3—40% to 50% Impairment

1. Roentgenographic appearance may be normal but is typically not
2. Dyspnea does not occur at rest but may occur during the normal activities of daily living. The patient cannot keep pace with other persons of the same age and built
3. FEV and FVC tests are 55 to 70% predicted value
4. Arterial saturation is usually 88% or greater at rest and after exercise

Class 4—60% to 90% Impairment

1. Roentgenographic appearance is usually abnormal
2. Dyspnea occurs during activities (eg, climbing one flight of stairs or walking 100 yards level surface); it may even occur at rest
3. FEV and FVC tests are less then 55% of predicted value
4. Arterial saturation is usually less than 88% at rest and after exercise

Pulmonary Surgery

1. **Lobectomy:** removal of a lobe of lung

2. **Pneumonectomy:** removal of portion of a lung

3. **Pleurectomy:** removal of the pleural sac

4. **Decortication:** removal of any restrictive membrane that limits pulmonary function from the surface of the lung

5. **Segmental resection:** excision of a segment of the lobe

6. **Wedge resection:** excision of a portion of a segment of the lobe

Pulmonary Terms

Apnea: absence of ventilation

Atelectasis: incomplete expansion of lung secondary to collapse of alveoli

Barrel chest: increased anterior-posterior diameter of the thorax

Bradypnea: slow respiratory rates, shallow abnormal depth; this is normal during sleep

Cyanosis: caused by low oxygen saturation; the skin has a bluish tint

Dyspnea: rapid rate, shallow depth (accessory muscle activity)

Flail chest: when two or more ribs are broken, the chest will move paradoxically during breathing

Hemothorax: blood in the pleural space

Hypercapnia: blood, CO_2 in arterial blood

Hyperpnea: rapid rate, increased depth

Hyperventilation: fast rate, increased depth

Hypoxia: fluid CO_2 in the blood, diminished availability of oxygen to the body tissue.

Orthopnea: difficulty breathing when in a position other than erect

Pes carinatum: the sternum protrudes forward and is abnormally prominent

Pectus excavatum: the sternum is abnormally depressed

Tachypnea: abnormally fast rate of breathing

Postural Drainage Contraindications (position head down)

1. Shunt
2. Head trauma
3. Cerebral hemorrhage
4. Cardiac condition in which increased venous return increases patient's chance of cardiac failure
5. Hypertension

Percussion Contraindications

1. Angina
2. Skin breakdown, wounds
3. Pneumothorax
4. Osteoporosis
5. Pulmonary emboli
6. Tumor

Chest Physical Therapy

Indications	Versus	Contraindications
Airway resistance		Cerebral edema
Poor ventilation		Aneurysm
Poor oxygenation		Severe hypertension
Fluid/mucus in airways		Cardiac complications
Poor chest mobility		Pulmonary edema
Dyspnea		Gastric regurgitation
Poor mucocilliary movements		Recent hemoptysis
Aspirations		Fractured rib
Pulmonary secretions		Pneumothorax
Atelectasis		Pulmonary embolus
		Open thoracic wounds
		Immediately after chest tube removal
		Osteoporosis

Patient Positions

Upper Lobes

1. Apical
   - Sitting upright
   - Percussion: between clavicle and scapula

2. Anterior
   - Supine, knees in a slightly flexed position, pillows underneath knees
   - Percussion: between clavicle and nipple

3. Posterior
   - Sitting in chair, patient leaning forward approximately 20° to 30°, resting on pillows
   - Percussion: top of shoulder blade

4. Left lingular
   - Right sidelying position, rotated backward one-quarter of a turn, foot of bed elevated 14 to 18 inches
   - Percussion: left side at nipple level

Middle Lobe

1. Right middle lobe
   - Left sidelying position, rotated backward half a turn, foot of bed elevated 14 inches, pillows under right hip
   - Percussion: right side at nipple level

Lower Lobes

1. Apical
   - Prone, pillows under stomach
   - Percussion: middle of back at inferior angle of scapula

2. Anterior
   - Supine, pillows under knees, foot of bed elevated 18 inches, chest tilted 20°
   - Percussion: anterior lower ribs

3. Posterior
   - Prone, pillows under the hips, foot of bed elevated 18 inches, chest tilted 20°
   - Percussion: posterior ribs, level should be close to the spine area

4. Lateral basal
   - Prone position, turned a half turn upward, foot of bed elevated 18 inches, chest tilted 20°
   - Percussion: lateral lower ribs

Pulmonary Therapy

Treatment Components

1. Airway Clearance Techniques
   - Cough: the patient is instructed to cough to assist in clearing secretions. The patient will perform coughing in the sitting position if possible.
   - Assisted cough: the therapist utilizes his or her hand/hands to assist the patient with coughing. The therapist will push inward and upward, forcing coughing and assisting the rapid exhalation of air.
   - Huff: the patient will deeply inhale and forcibly expel the air while saying "Ha, ha." This is affected in patients who have collapsed airways and cannot tolerate high intrathoracic pressure.
   - Forced expiratory technique: the therapist uses this technique with the patient to assist in the removal of peripheral secretions. The patient starts with diaphragmatic breathing, performs thoracic expansion exercises, controlled diaphragmatic breathing, inhales resting tidal volume, lastly contracts the abdominal muscles to produce forced expiratory huffs.
   - Tracheal stimulation: this technique is used for patients who cannot cough when asked. The therapist places his or her finger or thumb above the suprasternal notch. Then the therapist applies quick inward and downward pressure on the trachea to elicit the cough reflex.

2. Bagging
   - Purpose: to provide artificial ventilation, restore oxygen, and re-expand the lungs.
   - Technique: to coordinate with the patient's breathing pattern. Attach manual resuscitator bag to the oxygen source and then connect it to the tracheal tube. Squeeze bag rhythmically to deliver volume of air to patient. Patient expires passively.
   - Indications: before and after suctioning a patient who is not mechanically ventilated.

3. Breathing Exercises
   - Purpose: to assist with the removal of secretions, relaxation, and increase thoracic cage mobility, tidal volume, increase ventilation, and improve gas exchange.
   - Technique: teach patient to produce a full inspiration followed by a controlled expiration. Use hand placement for sensory feedback and lateral and diaphragmatic costale excursion. Use gentle pressure through exhalation breathing activity.
   - Indications: utilize with spontaneously breathing patients.

Breathing Exercises

1. Diaphragmatic Breathing
   - Purpose: to increase ventilation, improve gas exchange, improve chest wall mobility, and prevent pulmonary compromise.
   - Technique: position the patient semireclined. The therapist will place his or her hand over the subcostal angle of the patient's thorax, then apply gentle pressure when the patient exhales and increasing to firm pressure at the end of exhalation. The patient will then inhale and the therapist will instruct the patient to resist the therapist's hand on inhalation. The therapist will then release pressure so the patient can fully inhale.
   - Indications: post-trauma patients. Postoperative patients, obstructive lung disease, and restrictive lung disease.

2. Pursed Lip Breathing
   - Purpose: increase tidal volume, reduce the respiratory rate, reduce dyspnea, and facilitate relaxation.
   - Technique: patient will slowly inhale through nose or mouth and passively exhale through pursed lips.
   - Indications: obstructive disease and to get the patient who has an unproductive breathing pattern to relax.

3. Segmental Breathing
   - Purpose: to prevent pulmonary compromise, improve chest wall mobility, increase ventilation to hyperventilated lungs, and redistribute gas.

- Technique: position patient in a specific segment for postural drainage (eg, upright sitting). The therapist will apply gentle pressure over the thorax of the patient during exhalation. The pressure will increase to firm just prior to inspiration. The patient will breathe in against the therapist's resistance. The therapist will lastly release pressure, allowing the patient to take a full inspiration.
- Indications: post-trauma, incisional, pleuritic pain with decreased movement in the thorax.

4. Sustained Maximal Inspiration
   - Purpose: to increase inhaled volume, improve alveolar inflation, and restore functional residual capacity.
   - Technique: have the patient inspire slowly through the nose or pursed lips to maximal inspiration, hold for 3 seconds, and passively exhale the volume.
   - Indications: acute lobar collapse, acute post-trauma pain, and acute postoperative pain.

5. Coughing
   - Purpose: to remove secretions from the larger airways.
   - Technique: inspiration gasp followed by closing of the glottis. Contraction of expiration muscles followed by opening of the glottis.
   - Indications: utilize with spontaneously breathing patients.

6. Patient Mobilization
   - Purpose: to prevent injurious sequelae from bedrest and immobility and to reduce the rehabilitation time.
   - Technique: turn and passively position the patient, passive and active range of motion, exercises, sitting, standing, and ambulation.
   - Indications: use with all patients according to their diagnosis and tolerance.

7. Percussion
   - Purpose: utilized in addition to postural drainage to mobilize secretions.

- Technique: during inspiration and expiration, rhythmically clap cupped hands over bare skin or thin material covering the area of involved lung.
- Indications: when secretions are not adequately cleared from coughing, suctioning, or from breathing exercises and mobilization of the patient.

8. Postural Drainage
    - Purpose: through the assistance of gravity, the patient's retained secretions are mobilized.
    - Technique: position patient so the involved segmental bronchus is uppermost.
    - Indications: when secretions are not adequately cleared from coughing, suctioning, or from breathing exercises and mobilization of the patient.

9. Suctioning
    - Purpose: to remove secretions from the larger airways.
    - Technique: utilizing an aseptic technique, furnish supplemental oxygen. Gently insert a suction catheter, then apply suction while withdrawing catheter. Re-expand the lung with a mechanical ventilator or manually with a resuscitator bag attached to a tracheal tube.
    - Indications: tracheal suctioning is for use only with those patients who have an artificial airway.

10. Vibration
    - Purpose: utilized in addition to postural drainage to mobilize secretions.
    - Technique: only perform during expiration, intermittent chest wall compression over the area of the involved lung.
    - Indications: when secretions are not adequately cleared from coughing, suctioning, or from breathing exercises and mobilization of the patient.

Pulmonary Assessment

1. History
2. Patient interview
3. Vital signs
   - Blood pressure
   - Heart rate
   - Respiration
4. Observation
   - Patient's color
   - Edema
   - Digital clubbing
   - Breathing pattern
5. Palpation
6. Range of motion
7. Graded exercise test
8. Chest wall mobility
9. Auscultation
10. Percussion
11. Description of patient's cough
12. Posture
13. Psychosocial support
14. Strength
    - Abdominalis
    - Back muscles

Chapter Eleven
Clinical Disorders

Acquired Immunodeficiency Syndrome (AIDS)

- An immunodeficiency disease characterized by progressive destruction of T-cells and lymphocytes.
- The disease leaves patients highly susceptible to infections.
- HIV (human immunodeficiency virus) is a retrovirus that is unique because some of the cells will escape from the body's immune system.
- Some patients who have AIDS never become infected. Patients who have the disease have different rates of progression.
- **Treatment:** no known cure; different treatment combinations work differently in each patient and may slow progression of the disease or the disease may go into remission. Secondary infections are the leading cause of death. Special implications for physical therapy are the use of universal precautions for health care workers. Exercises for pain relief and prevention of muscle atrophy/strength/endurance are beneficial to patients. Breathing exercises, posture instructions, balance activities, and activities of daily living assessment are also potential physical therapy treatment areas.

Buerger's Disease

- Also called thromboangiitis obliterans.
- Results in inflammatory changes in arteries and veins.
- Diagnostic test in physical therapy is to place toes/foot in dependent position—will see rubor color; then place toes/foot above heart level—will see pallor color.
- **Treatment:** must stop smoking, avoid extreme temperatures, and avoid wearing tight clothing. Buerger's exercise protocol.

Cushing's Disease

- Metabolic disorder characterized by abnormally increased secretion of adrenocortical steroids. Caused by increased amounts of adreno-corticotrophic hormone (ACTH), secreted by the anterior lobe of the pituitary gland.
- Results in accumulation of fat and edema on the chest, upper back and face.
- Also called hyperadrenocorticism.
- **Treatment:** removal or destruction of adrenocortical steroids-secreting tissue, usually by surgical or radiologic procedures.

Deep Venous Thrombosis

- The formation of an abnormal blood clot in a deep vein.
- The danger is in the clot breaking free, resulting in a pulmonary embolus.
- Symptoms may vary; skin may appear cyanotic, warm, cold, or normal temperature.
- Pain, tenderness, and edema may be present.
- Superficial thrombophlebitis is not an emergency and does not require hospitalization.
- **Treatment:** typically consistsof warm compresses over the involved veins and anti-inflammatory drugs. Deep venous thrombosis treatment includes hospitalization, bed rest with elevated lower extremities and anticoagulants.

Diabetes Insipidus

- Disease involving the imbalance of water secondary to an antidiuretic hormone (ADH) secreted by the posterior lobe of the pituitary gland.
- This disease can be caused by injury or lack of functioning to the following: hypothalamus, posterior pituitary gland, and the neurohypophyseal track.
- This water imbalance results in excessive excretion of diluted urine.
- **Treatment:** no specific physical therapy intervention. Treatment is usually replacement of antidiuretic hormone with synthetic derivatives. Caution is for physical therapist to monitor patient's condition during treatment for high blood pressure, water intoxication, and seizures.

Diabetes Mellitus

- Results in carbohydrate intolerance.
- Patient is unable to produce a sufficient amount of insulin or, more commonly, develops peripheral resistance to a normal or increased amount of secreted insulin.
- Type I diabetes is considered insulin-dependent to prevent ketosis. This was previously called juvenile-onset diabetes.
- Type II diabetes is considered noninsulin dependent. Typically, this is adult-onset diabetes.
- Hypoglycemia symptoms include sweating, pallor skin color, headaches, dizziness, irritable and nervous mood, and patient is hungry and shaky.
- Hyperglycemia symptoms include flushed skin, dehydration, thirst, weakness, nausea, vomiting, and lethargic mood.
- **Treatment:** diet adjustment or insulin depending upon the severity of the disease. The goal of treatment is to maintain normal blood glucose levels. Special implications for the physical therapist include knowing the signs and symptoms of a patient going into a diabetic coma, hypoglycemia, or hyperglycemia. A therapist should be aware of how exercises affect a patient with diabetes mellitus. Physical therapist may also be involved with wound care in diabetics.

Hemophilia

- Heritatary disorder resulting in deficiency in the clotting factor. The results are a bleeding disorder that can result in small or large blood losses.
- Hemophilia type A is caused by a deficiency or absence of antihemophilia factor VIII.
- Hemophilia type B is caused by a deficiency of plasma thromboplastin.
- Hemarthrosis and muscle bleeds are of particular concern in physical therapy.
- **Treatment:** splinting, ice, rests, and elevation is needed in the acute stage. In chronic situations, joint protection, maintaining joint function, daily exercise for ROM, strength and endurance, ADL training, and use of appropriate splints and assistive devices.

Hepatitis

- Acute or chronic inflammation of the liver.
- May be caused by alcohol abuse, drug reactions, chemical reaction, or a virus.
- Hepatitis A is an acute infection acquired through contaminated water/food, or spread by saliva and feces. It does not lead to chronic hepatitis.
- Hepatitis B is the second major cause of cirrhosis in the United States. It is acquired through exposure to blood and infected body fluids.
- Hepatitis C is typically acquired through blood transfusion and 50% of cases progress to chronic hepatitis. It may also be acquired with needlesticks and intravenous drug usage.
- Hepatitis D is uncommon in the United States and is typically associated with drug addicts, sexually active teenagers, and patients receiving several transfusions. This type of hepatitis results in progression to chronic active hepatitis and death.
- Hepatitis E is rare in the United States and typically found in developing countries. Patients at risk are typically travelers. It does not progress to chronic hepatitis. Transmitted through contamination of water.
- **Treatment:** medical management depends on the type of hepatitis found and the extent of the liver damage.

Hernia

- A protrusion of an organ through an abnormal opening in the wall.
- Most common types are direct and indirect inguinal, femoral, incisional, and umbilical.
- The main reason for occurrence is a weakness in the abdominal muscles.
- Inguinal hernia is the most common type, involving 75% of all hernias.
- **Treatment:** supports and trusses can contain the hernia. Surgical intervention is necessary for correction.

Hodgkin's Disease

- A malignant disorder that results in progressive enlargement in lymph tissue.

- Symptoms include weight loss, low grade fever, anemia, night sweats, and leukocytosis.
- Common areas affected are the spleen, liver, and bone marrow.
- May be fatal, but typically 50% of patients have long-term remission.
- **Treatment:** radiotherapy and/or chemotherapy.

Huntington's Chorea

- Hereditary disease.
- Results in progressive mental deterioration.
- Characterized by irregular movements and tremors.
- Disease typically occurs during the fourth decade of life.
- Average survival rate is 15 years after diagnosis.
- **Treatment:** no specific physical therapy treatment, but symptoms may be alleviated or decreased through medication therapy.

Leukemia

- An abnormal form and amount of immature white blood cells in the bone marrow. The normal cells are replaced with malignant neoplasm, resulting in bone marrow failure.
- The cells are malignant and can overflow from the bone marrow into the peripheral circulation and progress to the lymph nodes, liver, and spleen.
- The three main symptoms are anemia, infection, and bleeding.
- Leukemia can be acute with a sudden onset and rapid progression of the disease.
- Leukemia may also be chronic with a slowly developing onset and progression.
- **Treatment:** chemotherapy, blood transfusion, antibiotics, bone marrow transplants, and supportive measures for pain and infections. Special considerations for physical therapy include awareness that patient is susceptible to infections and bleeding. Physical therapy treatments may include safety instructions because of patient weakness, education on pressure points and prevention of sores, and general range of motion and gentle stretching exercises depending on blood tests.

Marfan's Syndrome

- Hereditary resulting in elongation of the bones.
- Typical appearance is tall, lean person. The extremities are very long and feet and hands are greatly extended. Patient is usually over 6 feet tall.
- Disease will affect muscle, bone, ligaments, and skeletal structures.
- Problems include ligament laxity, lateral curvature of the spine, joint hypermobility, muscular underdevelopment, pes valgus, and genu recurvatum.
- **Treatment:** no specific physical therapy treatment. Orthosis may be utilized to assist with deformities.

Pancreatitis

- Serious inflammation of the pancreas; may be acute or chronic.
- It can result in the pancreas being digested by its own enzymes.
- Acute pancreatitis may be caused by alcoholism, medications, hereditary, trauma, peptic ulcers, viral infections, and post-surgical inflammation.
- Chronic pancreatitis is caused by structural or functional impairment of the pancreas.
- **Treatment:** medical management of acute pancreatitis consists of management of symptoms, as it typically subsides in several days. Chronic pancreatitis treatment is focused on prevention of further damage to the pancreas.

Psoriasis

- A chronic, inherited, reoccurring skin disease.
- Characterized by erythematous plaque covered with silvery scales on the skin.
- Fifteen to twenty percent of patients may develop psoriasis arthritis.
- **Treatment:** no known cure; physical therapy intervention is treatment with ultraviolet light.

Raynaud's Syndrome

- Caused by spasm in small blood vessels.

- Intermittent attacks of ischemia in the extremities.
- Common in the hands; may also be in the toes, ears, and nose.
- Results in intermittent attacks of blanching, cyanosis, and redness.
- The attacks may cause pain, numbness, burning, and tingling sensations.
- **Treatment:** vasodilators; avoid exposure to excessive temperatures, caffeine, and smoking. Education on protecting body from the elements and sometimes biofeedback.

Reflex Sympathetic Dystrophy

- Typically follows an injury (eg, a sprain or fracture).
- Injury results in damage to afferent pathways of sensory processing.
- Characterized by persistent pain above the normally accepted pain level.
- Initially injury will show swelling and increased tissue temperature.
- Later the skin will appear dry, shiny, and leathery.
- **Treatment:** contrast baths, electrical stimulation, range of motion.

Rheumatic Heart Disease

- Caused by rheumatic fever.
- Result is serious heart defects (valvular) and damage to the heart muscle.
- Heart murmurs present.
- Damage may result in permanent heart deformities.
- **Treatment:** no specific physical therapy. Medical management depends on significance of heart damage.

Scleroderma

- Result is a thickening of skin and subcutaneous tissues caused by new collagen formation.
- Most common in middle-age women.
- Serious if it affects the organs.
- Frequently it is accompanied by Raynaud's syndrome.
- **Treatment:** maintain range of motion, prevent contractures, and muscle strengthening.

Systemic Lupus Erythematosus

- Collagen vascular disorder.
- Primarily affects the connective tissue in the skin, joints, blood vessels, and internal organs.
- Inflammatory response seen.
- Characteristics are fever, butterfly rash, polyarthritis, vasculitis, pericarditis, and renal involvement.
- Women are more commonly affected—two to three times more then men.
- **Treatment:** medications, joint conservation techniques. Ultraviolet treatment is contraindicated.

Thrombus

- Formation of a clot from accumulation of fibrin, platelets, cellular elements of blood, and clotting factors.
- May be either blood or fat clot.
- Typically, the clot is attached to the interior wall of a vein or artery.
- **Treatment:** anticoagulant drug therapy.

Ulcer (Peptic) Disease

- A break in the protective mucus lining resulting in gastric acid going into the submucosal areas.
- Peptic ulcers involve proteolytic enzymes, which are the main component in the digestion process.
- Gastric ulcers are a type of peptic ulcer that affects the lining of the stomach.
- Duodenum ulcers are a type of peptic ulcer that occurs in the duodenum.
- Stress may also cause ulcers in varying degrees.
- **Treatment:** medical management utilizing drug therapy to promote healing, pain relief, and prevention of complications. Prevention of future ulcers may be helped through education on stress reduction. Surgical intervention is necessary in severe cases where there is perforation.

Chapter Twelve

Wound Care & Burns

Skin and Tissue

The skin is the largest organ of the body. Its functions include protective covering, regulation of body temperature, aiding in regulation of blood pressure, housing sensory receptors, and synthesizing various chemicals. The skin is composed of the following layers:

Epidermis

- Outer layer of the skin
- Layers are between 0.5 and 1.1 mm in thickness
- Contains striated squamous epithelium cells
- Functions to protect the underlying tissue against water loss, effects of harmful chemicals, and mechanical injury
- Location of the pores and the hair shafts

Dermis

- Binds the epidermis to underlying tissues
- Composed of fibrous connective tissue
- Contains nerves, nerve endings, glands, hair follicles, blood, and lymphatic vessels
- Functions with vitamin D production
- The following are contained in the dermis:
    - ✓ Ducts
    - ✓ Arrector pili muscles
    - ✓ Sebaceous glands
    - ✓ Nerves
    - ✓ Blood vessels

Subcutaneous Tissue

- A continuous layer of connective tissue beneath the dermis. It comprises an outer, normally fatty layer, and an inner, thin elastic layer
- Composed of adipose tissue
- Anchors the superficial tissue layers to the underlying tissue

Skin Response to Injury

Burns

- Minor burns will cause the blood vessels to dilate and the tissue surrounding the area to become red
- Response is localized to the injured area in small minor burns
- As burns become more severe in nature, blisters will form in the skin due to fluid being retained underneath the skin
- In severe burns, the protective skin layer will be removed. The wound may heal by filling in or skin grafts may be necessary
- Burns, depending upon the damage, will affect the following systems in the body, renal, respiratory, cardiovascular, gastrointestinal, pulmonary, and immune system.

Wound Healing Response

- There are three phases in the wound healing response: inflammatory, proliferation, and the remodeling.
- The inflammatory stage is where you see the cardinal signs of inflammation: calor (heat), rubor (redness), dolor (pain), and tumor (swelling).
- The blood vessels will dilate, becoming red and permeable. The vascular permeability allows fluids to enter the damaged tissues. This is what causes the redness and pain response.
- The proliferation stage results in exudation of the fluid, clustering of leukocytes in the vessel walls, phagocytosis of debri, and deposits of fibrin.
- The remodeling stage results in migration of fibroblasts and development of new normal cells.

Classification of Ulcers

Stages

1. **Stage one:** destruction is limited to the epidermis and redness may be noted. Nonblanchable erythemia of the skin and a heralding lesion of skin ulceration.
2. **Stage two:** involvement of the epidermis, dermis, and subcutaneous fat; redness, edema, blistering, and hardening of the tissue may be noted. The ulcer is superficial and may appear as an abrasion, blister, or a shallow crater.
3. **Stage three:** full thickness of dermis is involved, and undermining of the deeper tissues may extend down to the underlying fascia. The ulcer is a deep crater that may or may not involve the undermining tissues.
4. **Stage four:** full thickness involves penetrating to the fascia with possible muscle involvement, and there is usually bone destruction.

Types of Ulcers

Arterial Insufficiency Ulcers

Occur secondary to arteriosclerosis obliterans, often in diabetics. Peripheral pulses are weak or absent. Bruits may be heard via stethoscope over peripheral vessels. Bruits are sounds of blood turbulence as a result of narrow vessels. Limb elevation will result in pallor. The dependent position (down) will cause rubor. The ulcers that may form are usually located on the lateral malleolus and toes. Can be very deep and painful. Bed rest with the head of the bed moderately elevated, no smoking, wound care and protective environment are conservative ways of managing these wounds. No external compression is used.

Venous Insufficiency Ulcers

Occur secondary to venous thrombosis, varicose veins, and other venous problems. Peripheral pulses usually are good and edema is present. The ulcers are usually located on the medial side of the ankle. The surrounding skin may be pigmented and indurated. They are often painless and may be extensive but not deep. They can endure for decades. Elevation and compression to control edema is vital. Unna's boot, custom-fitted elastic stockings, and intermittent compression therapy can be helpful. Wound care is performed, however, whirlpool is not helpful. Exercise is permissible if support garments are worn and the part is elevated after exercising.

Diabetic Ulcers

Diabetic ulcers occur as a result of improper glucose metabolism, resulting in a diminished vascular system. Sensory neuropathy may also occur in diabetics, leading to a loss of sensation. Diabetic ulcers result because of repetitive stress and pressure on the skin lacking sensory input. The lack of sensory input results in the patient not protecting the injured area, then the subcutaneous and cutaneous break down. A common area of ulcers to occur is over bony areas, like the medial malleolus, lateral malleolus, and greater trochanter. Diabetic ulcer treatment depends on additional factors outside of physical therapy treatment plans. The patient's nutritional balance, insulin control, glucose levels, and exercise level all integrate with the healing process. These factors must also be working for optimal wound healing in conjunction with physical therapy treatments.

Location of Ulcers

Ulcers may be caused by prolonged pressure over bony areas or possibly from a lack of healing in an area. For example, in a diabetic patient, they most likely occur over bony areas, such as the medial malleolus, lateral malleolus, and greater trochanter. The following are risk factors for a pressure ulcer: friction between surfaces, external pressure on an area, two layers sliding against each other in opposite directions, and softening caused by excessive moisture. There are additional risk factors for patient's who have restricted mobility. As a result of restricted mobility, the risk factors are contractures, obesity, and loss of sensation, edema, and increased muscle tone.

Evaluation of the Wound

When evaluating the wound it is important to note the following:
* History of patient
* General health
* Vital signs—pulses and blood pressure
* Observation of wound
* Cultures of wound
* Determine the size, depth, and shape
* Color of wound and surrounding tissue
* Evaluation of wound drainage
* Location of wound
* Temperature of wound
* Texture of wound
* Vascular examination
* Girth measurements
* Auscultation of arteries
* Percussion test
* Trendelenburg test
* Homan's sign
* Sensory test

Treatment of the Wound

1. Cleansing the wound to promote healing. Whirlpool may be utilized with wounds to remove loosely attached debri and clean the wound bed. Whirlpools should be set up with a sterile technique. Additives, such as antibacterial agents, may be utilized depending on the type of wound. All staff members should wear protective barriers.

2. Debridement of the wound of necrotic or damaged tissue. The necrotic tissues obstruct the formation of granulation and epithelial cells from migrating across the wound. The debridement may consist of a whirlpool with agitation directed at the wound. Debridement may also take place using a scalpel, scissors, and forceps. This is only utilized when it is clear that the tissue is devitalized.

3. Dressings that are removed from the patient should be placed in a biohazard container as per facility policy.

4. Patient's dressing should be reapplied after treatment, utilizing sterile techniques and protective barriers.

5. Pressure-relieving devices, such as foam padding, may be utilized to protect the wound from further pressure and deterioration.
6. Teach weight shifting or turning schedules to the patients, family, and staff for home education programs.
7. Exercises can increase circulation to the area to promote healing. Exercises can also be utilized to prevent contracutres, increase muscle strength, and decrease edema.
8. Oxygen, ultrasound, and electrical stimulation may be utilized to increase wound healing.
9. A physician may utilize surgery to remove excessive necrotic and debri tissue.
10. If possible, restoring normal function to the tissue is the final goal.

Prevention of Wounds

1. In diabetic cases, provide the patient with the proper education. Also, early intervention will aid in preventing the ulcer from entering the later stages.
2. Check skin frequently for red spots.
3. Patients at risk should at least have a daily skin inspection.
4. Skin should be thoroughly cleaned at the time it is soiled, prevent infection through proper cleaning as soon as possible.
5. Immobile patients should be placed on a frequent turning schedule.
6. Proper position of the bedridden patient and frequent repositioning every 2 hours.
7. Pressure-reducing devices should be utilized. Wheelchair patients should have a doughnut type device. In bed, positioning devices should include pillows and foam wedges. Bedridden patients should use pressure-reducing surfaces, foam, gel, air, or water mattress.
8. Transferring techniques should emphasize reducing friction through utilization of a slide board, trapeze, and hydraulic lifts.
9. At a minimum, maintain current range of motion and mobility. If the patient has rehabilitation potential, try to increase the activity level and mobility.
10. Environment for patients should be stable with little fluctuation to cold/hot temperatures or humidity that creates dry skin.
11. Utilization of lubricants, like creams, can decrease friction between surfaces sliding on one another.

Classification of Burns

Superficial burn

- Minimal thickness
- Affects the epidermis only
- Skin appears red
- Skin surface is dry
- Slight pain
- Minimal edema
- No blistering
- Healing with no scarring

Superficial Partial-Thickness Burn

- Affects the epidermis and possibly the superficial part of the dermis
- Severe pain
- Considerable edema
- Mottled appearance
- Blister formations intact
- Healing with minimal or no scarring

Deep Partial-Thickness Burn

- Damage to entire epidermis, as well as severe damage to the dermis
- Broken blisters
- Wound color a mixed red or waxy white color
- Severe pain or possible loss of pain if nerve endings are damaged
- Moderate edema
- Healing occurs with hypertrophic scarring and keloids

Full-Thickness Burns

- Complete destruction of the entire epidermis and dermis
- Possible damage to subcutaneous fat layer
- Hard parchment-like eschar formation
- No pain
- No blisters
- Severe edema
- White leathery appearance
- Healing tissue only occurs at the edges of the wound requiring skin grafting

Subdermal Burns

- Complete destruction of the epidermis, dermis, and fat layers
- May damage the bone and muscle
- Typically as a result of prolong contact with a flame, chemical or electricity
- Extensive surgery is required
- Sometimes amputation is necessary

Rule of Nines

This allows the therapist to determine the percentage of the body burned. The rule of nines was developed by Lund and Brower. The rule of nines is based on dividing the body into sections, which represent 9% or a multiple of 9%. Each area of the body is assigned a specific value, as listed in the following chart:

Body Area	Adults	Children
Head—anterior	4.5%	18%
Head—posterior	4.5%	
Arm—anterior	4.5%	9%
Arm—posterior	4.5%	
Leg—anterior	9%	14%
Leg—posterior	9%	
Chest	18%	18%
Back	18%	18%
Genitals	1%	1%

Graft and Flap Types

Advancement flap: a local flap where adjacent skin is moved to cover the burn without detaching the flap from its existing site.

Allograft: may also be called a homograft; a graft is taken from a donor who is the same species but not identical to the patient. See homograft definition.

Autograft: skin taken from a part of the burn victim's own body.

Biosynthetic graft: a graft that is a combination of collagen and synthetics.

Delayed graft: a graft that is partially elevated, then replaced. It is replaced so that it can be moved to another site.

Free flap: skin tissue that is moved to another site where vascular reconnection is made. The moved skin tissue may also include blood vessels.

Full-thickness graft: consists of all layers of skin but no subcutaneous fat.

Heterograft or xenograft: skin taken from another species. Most often pigskin dressing to speed healing. Temporary grafts.

Homograft: human skin from a donor (often cadaver skin is used).

Isologous graft: donor and patient are genetically identical.

Local flap: movement of skin to an adjacent site. Part of the flap will remain attached to retain its blood supply.

Mesh graft: the donor's skin is cut away from the mesh so it can cover a larger surface area.

Myocutaneous flap: the flap consists of muscle, patent blood vessels, skin, and subcutaneous fat.

Sheet graft: the donor's skin is applied without changing the recipient's site.

Split-thickness skin graft: autograft that is one-half thickness of skin.

Test-tube graft: a biopsy providing epidermal cells that are cultured into smooth sheets of skin. These sheets of skin are then grafted onto the burn area. This is a new procedure utilized for burns that cover the entire body.

Z–plasty: a simple form of the rotational flab where a section of skin is incised on three sides and pivoted to cover the injured area.

Treatment of Burn Patients

1.   Sterile whirlpool in order to promote healing. This is done to control infection and aid in loosening the necrotic tissue, making debridement easier. Sterile towels and dressing must also be used post-whirlpool. It is extremely important to maintain a faultless sterile technique so that no cross-infections occur.
2.   Reduce dependent edema formation and promote venous return.
3.   Proper positioning and splinting to control contractures and edema.
4.   Passive range of motion and stretching exercises.
5.   Closure of the wound. Grafting as necessary. Physician may utilize medications to assist in controlling infections and pain. Pain relievers may be given 45 minutes prior to treatment to assist with the pain from the treatment program.
6.   Active range of motion progressing from therapist assistance to resistive exercise as tolerated.
7.   Pressure garments for reducing edema and scar formation.
8.   Massage to reduce scarring and tissue contracutres.
9.   Increase strength, range of motion, and functioning.
10.   Promote independence in activities of daily living and self-care.
11.   Proprioceptive and sensation exercises.
12.   Referral to counseling or support services (social worker, occupational therapy and vocational counselor) as necessary.
13.   Instructions in a home care program to promote burn healing, prevention of infection, prevention of edema and scar formation, and maintainence of normal joint function.

Burn Positioning to Prevent Contractures

Affected area	Positioning
Ankle/foot	Neutral. May use padded footboard or ankle position devices
Knee	Extension with posterior splint, toes pointing toward the ceiling
Hip	Extension/abduction/neutral rotation and toes pointing toward the ceiling.
Shoulder	Abduction/flexion/external rotation— may use clavicle strap or abduction axillary splint
Axillary region	Arm abducted to 90° to 110°
Elbow	Extension and supination. Elbow splinting position in extension with slight degree of elbow flexion
Wrist	Wrist placed in extension with a hand splint
Metacarpophalangeal (MCP) joint	MCP flexion at 90° with a hand splint
Proximal or distal inter-phalangeal joint (PIP/DIP)	PIP and DIP are placed in extension with a hand splint
Thumb	Thumb abduction with a hand splint
Web spaces	Finger abduction utilizing web spaces, gauze, or foam
Burn claw hand	MP flexion (70°), IP extension, thumb opposition, wrist extended (15°).
Anterior neck	Hyperextension, cervical brace, no pillows, may have a small towel beneath the cervical spine to promote extension
Posterior neck	Neutral position with no pillow
Circumferential neck involvement	Neutral position toward extension with no pillow

Chapter Thirteen

Diagnostic Testing

Arterial Blood Gas

The oxygen and carbon dioxide in arterial blood is measured by various methods to assess the adequacy of ventilation and oxygenation, as well as the acid base status. The normal pH of arterial blood is 7.4.

Bronchoscopy

Visual examination of the tracheobronchial tree utilizing a standard rigid, tubular metal bronchoscope or a narrower, flexible fiberoptic bronchoscope. The patient should have fasted and is typically sedated before the examination.

Cerebral Angiography

An x-ray procedure for visualizing the vascular system of the brain. Radiopaque contrast material is injected into the carotid, subclavian, brachial, or femoral artery with x-rays at specific intervals.

Computed Tomography (CT Scan)

An x-ray technique that produces a film representing a detailed cross-section of tissue structure. CT scan employs a narrowly collimated beam of x-rays that rotates in a continuous 360° motion around the patient. The image is created by computer using multiple readings of the patient in cross-sectional slices. This is a noninvasive and painless procedure for the patient.

Echoencephalogram

A recording produced by an echoencephalograph, which uses ultrasound to study the intracranial structures of the brain.

Electrocardiogram (ECG)

A graphic record produced by an electrocardiograph, which is a device used for recording the electric activity of the myocardium. It is used to detect abnormal transmission of the cardiac impulse through the conductive tissues of the muscle. The patient is positioned supine and must remain still. Leads are affixed to certain anatomical points on the patient's chest with adhesive gel that promotes transmission of the electric impulse to the recording device.

Electroencephalography (EEG)

The process of recording brainwave activity. Electrodes are attached to various areas of the patient's head. The patient must refrain from talking or moving and must remain still. The test is used to diagnose seizure and brainstem disorders, focal lesions, and impaired consciousness.

Electromyogram (EMG)

A record of the intrinsic electric activity in a skeletal muscle is obtained by applying surface electrodes or by inserting a needle electrode into the muscle. The physician observes electrical activity with an oscilloscope and a loudspeaker. EMGs also measure electric potentials induced by voluntary muscular contraction.

Evoked Potential (EP)

A tracing of a brainwave measured on the surface of the head at various places. The evoked potential is elicited by a specific stimulus, which may affect the visual, somatosensory, and auditory pathways, producing a characteristic brainwave pattern.

Fluoroscopy

A technique in radiology for visually examining a part of the body or the function of an organ using a fluoroscope. This technique delivers immediate serial images.

Lumbar Puncture (LP)

The introduction of a hollow needle and stylet into the subarachnoid space of the lumbar portion of the spinal canal at the third and fourth lumbar vertebrae. The patient is placed in a lateral recumbent position, with the back as near to the edge of the bed as possible. The legs should be flexed with the thighs flexed on the abdomen. Head and shoulders should be bent down, curving the spine convexly to grant the greatest amount of space between the vertebrae.

Magnetic Resonance Imaging (MRI)

MRI is medical imaging that utilizes nuclear magnetic resonance as a source of energy. This procedure is noninvasive and painless for the patient. It allows for three-dimensional viewing and high resolution.

Myelography

A radiographic process by which the spinal cord and the spinal subarachnoid space are viewed and photographed. A contrast medium is introduced. This test is used to identify spinal lesions.

Nerve Conduction Velocity (NCV)

Refers to the maximum nerve conduction velocity, which is the speed with which an electrical impulse can be transmitted through excitable tissue.

Ultrasound Imaging

The use of high-frequency sound waves to take images of internal structures. This is performed by measuring and recording the reflection of the high frequency sound waves.

Ventriculography

An x-ray examination of the head after an injection of air or other contrast medium into the cerebral ventricles, or an x-ray examination of a ventricle of the heart after the injection of a radiopaque contrast medium.

X-Ray (Roentgen Ray)

Electromagnetic radiation of shorter wavelength than visible light. It is produced when electrons traveling at high speed strike certain materials. It can be used to investigate the integrity of structures, to therapeutically destroy dead tissue, and to make photographic images for diagnostic purposes.

Chapter Fourteen
Psychology

Common Disorders

Affective Psychosis

- Psychotic reaction
- Mental disorder of organic or emotional origin
- Characterized by extreme derangement or disorganization of personality
- Accompanied by severe depression, agitation, regressive behavior, illusions, delusions, and hallucinations
- Usually requires hospitalization because the patient is incapable of functioning in society

Alzheimer's Disease

- Chronic, progressive, widespread deterioration of the cerebrum
- Intellectual decline, loss of memory, confusion, anxiety, depression, loss of reasoning
- As disease progresses, there may be some motor impairment, gait problems, or contractures
- Consistency of treatment and redirection to another task if the patient becomes frustrated are considerations during treatment

Conversion Disorder

- May also be known as hysteria
- A response to severe emotional stress, resulting in loss or impairment of some motor or sensory function
- Often connected with the nervous system, resulting in problems

with vision, sensation, hearing, or motor disturbances like hemiplegia, paraplegia, quadriplegia, tics, or tremors
- There is no known organic cause for this

Depression

- A feeling of sadness or helplessness
- Patient typically has little drive for activity or achievement. Patient may cry easily and there may be an eating disorder
- May be altered with the assistance of medication. The therapist needs to take a positive attitude, build in successful treatment experiences for the patient, and involve the patient in making choices about the types of treatments available

Hypochondria

- An overconcern with physical health
- Extreme anxiety about health
- May have no physiological basis for health problems

Mania

- Type of psychosis
- State of mental disorder
- Person exhibits a behavior of euphoria

Manic-Depressive Psychosis

- Wide swings in behavior between periods of euphoria and extreme depression
- Patient may be suicidal
- Bipolar disorder

Neurosis

- Inefficient way of coping with anxiety
- Involves the use of the unconscious defense mechanism
- An emotional disturbance

Obsessive-Compulsive Neurosis

- Neurotic condition
- Characterized by the inability to resist the intrusion of persistent, irrational thoughts, ideas, or fears

Obsessive-Compulsive Personality

- Type of personality disorder
- Characterized by an uncontrollable need to perform certain acts or rituals
- When the acts become irrational, they interfere with acts of living in society

Paranoia

- A psychotic state or disorder
- Patient has delusions of persecution or grandiosity
- Patient is typically suspicious in all situations with all people

Psychopathy

- Patient may also be called a sociopath
- An antisocial personality disorder
- Characterized by behavior patterns that lack moral and ethical standards

Psychosis

- Mental disorder of organic or emotional origin
- Characterized by an extreme derangement or disorganization of personality
- Accompanied by depression, agitation, and hallucinations
- Person often requires hospitalization and cannot function in society

Schizophrenia

- Recognized through odd and bizarre behaviors
- Thoughts are distorted
- Very suspicious of others
- Withdrawl into fantasy life
- Patient may be destructive or impulsive

Suicide

- Occurs as a result of feeling hopeless or helpless
- Patient experiences a sense of rejection
- May be prevented. Encourage patient to discuss feelings and refer to appropriate services

Common Terms

Behavior Modification

- Attempt to change the patient's attitude toward pain, grooming or appearance, and willingness to participate in therapy
- Reinforce or reward healthy, positive, and socially appropriate behavior

Defense Mechanism

- An unconscious response by which the ego is protected from anxiety, guilt, or shame.
    - ✓ Denial: refusal to recognize external reality
    - ✓ Repression: inability to recall past events
    - ✓ Displacement: transferring an emotion to a substitute emotion
    - ✓ Reaction formation: behavior that is exactly opposite of what is expected
    - ✓ Projection: attributing your own unwanted trait to another

Empathy

- Capacity to understand what your patient is experiencing from his or her perspective
- Empathy helps you to better understand the meaning of the illness or disability, thereby strengthening your working relationship as you treat the patient

Grief Process

- Patients who lose body parts, functions, or clarity of mental processing may go through some, or all, of the following stages of grieving:
    - ✓ Denial
    - ✓ Anger
    - ✓ Bargaining
    - ✓ Depression
    - ✓ Acceptance

Perseveration

- Patient continues to repeat a movement, word, or expression
- Often accompanies a head injury or brain damage from stroke

Placebo

- Inactive treatment given for potential research benefit
- Used in experimental drug studies to compare the effects of the inactive substance with those of the experimental drug

Chapter Fifteen

Oncology

Terms

Benign Tumors

A tumor that is localized, slow growing, and does not invade other tissue or metastasize in other body sites. It may grow in size to become harmful if it impairs functions of the body.

Cancer Staging

A system for describing the extent of a malignant tumor and its metastases. It is utilized to plan a treatment program and predict a prognosis. The American Joint Committee on Cancer recommends staging cancer as follows: stage one is the primary tumor, stage two involves the primary tumor and lymph nodes, and stages three involves the primary tumor, lymph nodes, and metastases in other areas.

Cancerous Malignancies

A neoplasm characterized by uncontrolled growth of neoplastic cells. The cells tend to invade surrounding tissue and metastasize to other body sites. Malignant cells are present.

Carcinoma

A malignant epithelial neoplasm that invades surrounding tissue and metatisizes to other body sites. Most commonly in the skin, large intestine, lungs, stomach, prostrate, cervix, or breast. Tumor is firm, irregular, and nodular.

Lymphoma

A disorder of a tumor or neoplasm in the lymphoid tissue. Examples include Hodgkin's disease, lymphatic leukemia, adenolymphoma, and Burkitt's lymphoma. Usually malignant but may be benign in rare cases. Characterized by enlarged lymph node(s).

Malignant Tumors

A tumor whose growth may cause death and tends to become worse over time. The tumor will invade surrounding tissue and metastasize to distant sites.

Neoplasm

Any abnormal growth of new tissue; it may be benign or malignant. The new tissue serves no purpose and may cause harm by competing for blood supply.

Oncology

The branch of medicine that studies tumors and cancerous malignancies.

Sarcoma

A malignant neoplasm of soft tissue; presents as painless swelling. The tumors are vascular and usually highly invasive. Tumors occur 40% in lower extremities, 20% in upper extremities, 20% in the trunk, and 20% in the head, neck, or retroperineuma.

Tumors

Characterized by progressive, uncontrolled proliferation of cells. A tumor may be localized, invasive, benign, or malignant. A tumor may be named by the location, the person who first identified this type of tumor, and/or cellular makeup.

Treatment Options

Surgery

- Surgical removal or resection of tissue as allowed by the growth and metastases in other areas.
- Tumor may be completely or partially removed or the entire area may be resected.
- For example, a radical mastectomy to treat breast cancer is the surgical removal of the entire breast. A dissection is the removal of tissue in an area surrounding the operative site.
- Symptoms may include weakness after surgery, soreness, limited range of motion, and edema.

Radiation Therapy

- Utilizing radioactive substances in the treatment of the disease.
- May be utilized prior to surgery to attempt to decrease the tumor size as an option to surgery or postoperatively.
- A radiation oncologist is a physician who specializes in the treatment of cancer through radiation.
- Radiation therapy may cause sickness. Volume of radiation and length of exposure and treatment area determine the severity of sickness.
- Symptoms may include headaches, nausea, vomiting, diarrhea, and anorexia.

Chemotherapy

- Treatment with chemical agents to destroy the cancer cells.
- The chemical agents function to decrease the cell's ability to replicate and destroy cancer cells.
- There are many different chemical agents available, and the physician determines the most appropriate. This could be based on the latest research, if a patient is in a clinical study, location and type of cancer, stage of cancer, and side effects to patient. Side effects vary with type of agents utilized.
- Drugs may be prescribed in conjunction with chemotherapy to prevent side effects, and reduce or assist with symptoms after chemotherapy.

Evaluation, Treatment, and Precautions

Initial Evaluation

Depends on the type, location, and staging of cancer. The evaluation could include muscle weakness, endurance level, range of motion, ability to perform activities of daily living (ADLs), gait evaluation, sensation, and safety of patient.

Treatment Options

Vary with the type, location, and treatment of cancer. Some examples include:

- Education of the patient and family to treatment protocols and procedures, and disease effects on the patient from a physical therapy perspective.
- Development of treatment plans: long- and short-term goals with patient/family.
- Patient and family should be aware of the risk of falling secondary to weakness. Provide home safety assessment.
- Development and increased ability to perform ADLs and functional abilities.
- Referral to support groups and other health care team members.
- Increased activity to tolerance, conditioning, and muscle strengthening.
- Teaching gait and ADLs techniques to patient and family to increase safety.
- Patient position during and after treatment to prevent pressure sores or contractures.
- Modalities as appropriate (eg, long course of treatment in a hospital bed may cause neck and back pain).
- Therapeutic exercises as tolerated, depending on condition. For example, the same patient above may benefit from the Williams/McKenzie exercise for back and neck pain.
- Home program education with family/patient to continue therapy at home.

Precautions

- Tumors in certain locations (eg, bone tumors may cause weakness to bone area, or lower or upper extremities).
- Cancer treatments may affect cardiac and respiratory causing side effects; therefore, cardiac/respiratory systems should be monitored in physical therapy.
- Exercise levels may be decreased and fatigue may occur.
- Infection levels for the patient may be sensitive, watch for any open wounds, and use sterile precautions. Wear a mask when treating a patient if you have a cold or infection.
- Safety of patients, as they may have decreased balance, numbness, and/or neuropathy in extremities.

Chapter Sixteen

Obstetrics & Gynecology

Physiological Changes During Pregnancy

- Most uterine weight gain is during week 20. The average weight gain is typically 20 to 30 pounds.
- No specific neurological disorders result solely from pregnancy.
- The renal system must expand and a common complaint in early stages of pregnancy is the need to go to the bathroom very frequently. Weakness in the pelvic floor walls might result in stress incontinence.
- Respiratory changes result in widening of the thoracic cage, progressive elevation of the diaphragm, and the center part of the diaphragm becomes flat. Breathing patterns become more costal than abdominal because of the elevation of the diaphragm. Hyperventilation and dyspnea may occur during exercise.
- Cardiovascular system changes result in increased blood volume, increased heart rate, cardiac output, decreased arterial blood pressure at the end of the first trimester and throughout pregnancy.
- Gastrointestinal functions change because of hormones and structural changes. Changes may include vomiting or nausea, heartburn, minor abdominal pains, and lactose intolerance.
- Metabolic changes in carbohydrates may result in pregnancy diabetes.
- Musculoskeletal changes:
  1. Postural changes may result in cervical and/or lumbar lordosis, forward head, and kyphosis.
  2. Hormone release of relaxin results in ligament laxity. This most commonly involves the sacroiliac joint and hypermobility.

3. Abnormal wall and pelvic floor muscular weakness. Diastasis recti abdominis may occur, resulting in lateral separation of the rectus abdominis.
4. Back pain occurs as a result of the ligament laxity and weakness of abdominal muscles.

- Balance changes from the pregnancy result in the center of gravity being shifted forward.
- Varicose veins may be a result of pregnancy causing pain in the lower extremities.
- Gait pattern typically reveals a waddling gait.

Treatment Options

1. First the physical therapist needs to be aware of precautions in treatment program planning.
   - Avoid exercises that strain the pelvic floor muscles.
   - Avoid exercises that strain the abdominal muscles.
   - Avoid deep heating modalities and agents.
   - Have the patient avoid holding her breath during exercises so as not to increase interthoracic pressure.
   - Avoid positions that place the buttocks higher then the chest.
   - Avoid exercises that result in abdominal compression.
   - Avoid stretching that involves the hip flexors and areas of ligament laxity.
2. Transcutaneous electrical nerve stimulation (TENS) may be utilized to assist with pain.
3. A sacroiliac support belt and/or an orthosis may assist in support and help with back pain.
4. Superficial heat and moist hot packs may be utilized to assist with muscle relaxation and pain.
5. Gait instructions to walk avoiding an abducted gait, decreasing the waddling gait pattern.
6. Stretching exercise for postural correction and muscular relaxation. Exercises are modified (eg, single knee to chest stretching, patient should be supported with pillows or towel rolls and sidelying).
7. Modified curl-ups for abdominal wall strengthening.
8. Teach proper body mechanics.
9. Pelvic floor exercises and pelvic stabilization exercises.

10. Postural exercises for stretching and strengthening.
11. Teach the patient to monitor her own vital signs during exercise and activities of daily living.
12. Teach ankle pumps and elevated support positions of lower extremities to assist with edema and varicose veins.
13. Utilize elastic stockings for assistance with varicose veins.
14. Relaxation techniques, breathing exercise, meditation, and yoga.

Chapter Seventeen
Geriatrics

Changes in Aging

Cardiovascular System

- Loss of arterial elasticity
- Increase in peripheral resistance
- Systolic blood pressure increases with age secondary to decreased compliance of the blood vessels
- Decline in cardiac output
- The capacity of circulation to adopt to changes in body positioning decreases
- Decreased myocardial contractility and heart valves may stiffen
- Decreased cardiac output, 40% decline of overall resting cardiac output between third and seventh decade of life
- Decreased stroke volume
- Difficulty in meeting demands for increased cardiac output secondary to maximum heart rate decreasing
- Diminished supply of oxygenated blood, causing fatigue
- Decreased nourishment to vital organs, edema, and impaired waste removal
- After exertion, more time is needed to return to normal cardiac functioning.
- Some elderly people experience increased arrhythmia as conduction through nodal tissues slows
- Pacemaker's cells of the ventricle decline
- Automatic function of Purkinje network slows

Pulmonary System

- Decrease in vital capacity and forced expiratory volume (FEV); FEV can decline 20 to 40 ml per year
- Decreased strength of respiratory muscles
- Stiffening of chest wall
- Loss of bone matrix in the thoracic cage
- More vulnerable to respiratory illnesses
- Decreased elastic recoil of the lungs
- Decreased elasticity of the bronchial walls
- Decrease in rate of oxygen consumed and decreased oxygen delivery, reducing capacity to consume oxygen
- Increased ventilation
- Perfusion mismatch in the exchange of oxygen and carbon dioxide between the lungs
- Reduced ability to cough and breathe deeply
- Increased thinning of alveolar walls
- Decreased inspiratory muscle strength
- Increased mucus layer thickening
- Greater susceptibility to respiratory disease

Skeletal System

- Vertebral column becomes more compressed, shorter, disc atrophy, and less flexibility
- Increased calcification and ossification of ligaments and elastic fibers in cartilage
- Bone mass decreases
- Bone looses resilience and becomes lighter
- Increased sensitivity to bone fractures
- Increased susceptibility to osteoporosis
- Increased anterior/posterior diameter of the thoracic spine
- Increased susceptibility to hip and knee degeneration
- Stiffness of joints as a result of the degenerative process in the synovium
- Stiffness when going from sit to stand or in weightbearing positions
- Skeletal changes in the temporal mandibular joints; loss of teeth can decrease the ability to eat and can affect speech

Muscular System

- Decreased muscle mass
- Decreased endurance and increased muscle fatigue
- Increase in interstitial fluid, collagen, and intracellular fat
- Loss of muscle elasticity
- Articular cartilage tissue water content decreases
- Stiffening of capsules and ligaments
- Increased formation of collagen fibers and loss of elastic fibers
- Prolongation of contraction tone, latency period, and relaxation time
- Enzymes that repair damage are unable to be replaced and repaired effectively
- Decreased endurance, the ability and amount of the enzymes involved in energy metabolism become degraded

Nervous System

- Brain weight decreases during the aging process
- Increased lipofuscin pigment in neurons
- Nerve conduction velocity decreases
- Sleep patterns change duration of deep sleep levels decreases and number of arousals from sleep increases
- Central temperature regulation functions become impaired, causing the elderly to be more susceptible to hyperthermia and hypothermia
- Degeneration of the integrative system
- Decrease in Purkinje cells of the cerebellum
- Atrophy of the medullary olives
- Trunk instability
- Losses in the vestibular, proprioceptive, kinesthetic, and visual mechanisms
- Postural instability
- Memory loss as a result of impaired neuronal function, debranching, shortening within the cortex, marked changes in prefrontal, temporal, and hippocampus

Endocrine and Metabolic Systems

- Adrenal cell degeneration, which can result in elevated blood sugar levels and increased glucose intolerance

- Thyroid activity decreases
- Metabolic energy decreases
- Liver tends to get smaller in measurement in advanced aging
- Body burns fewer calories
- Lower immunity; hormones with the immune system decline

Senses

- Kinesthesia—the ability to perceive changes in body orientation and position in space declines with aging
- Vestibular senses decrease, which can result in accidental falls
- Vibration sensitivity declines
- Temperature sensations decline as well as the ability to maintain constant body temperature
- Visual field may decline, causing difficulty with perception and slower responses to tasks involving spatial ability; acuity and accommodation slow with steady decline
- Hearing loss may occur, which may be dangerous (eg, inability to hear approaching automobile)

Assessment/Screening

1. Home safety
2. Exercise level/current activity level
3. Nutritional problems
4. Observations
   - Does patient appear dehydrated?
   - Difficulty breathing?
   - Skin color
   - Weight/height observations
5. Overall health/history
6. Medications
7. Vital signs
   - Blood pressure
   - Respiratory rate
   - Pulses
   - Heart rate
8. Musculoskeletal
   - Motor planning/mobility
   - Balance/dynamic and static

- Range of motion/goniometry
- Flexibility
- Muscular endurance
- Muscular strength/manual muscle testing
9. Cognitive functioning
10. Coordination
    - Equilibrium
    - Nonequilibrium
11. Vascular testing
    - Girth measurements
    - Homan's sign
    - Reactive hyperemia
    - Ischemia and rRubor test
12. Skin integrity
13. Sensory abilities
    - Protective sensation
    - Discriminatory sensations
14. Posture
    - Posterior view
    - Lateral views
    - Anterior view
15. Gait
    - Cadence
    - Width of base of support
    - Length of step
    - Center of gravity
    - Arm swing
    - Observation of gait deviations
    - Amount of assistance necessary
16. Family status/support system
17. Sample treatment programs
    - **Cardiovascular:** aerobic exercises to increase oxygen uptake from blood.
    Examples: walking, biking, dancing, and swimming
    - **Muscular:** increase muscular endurance
    Examples: walking, swimming, and water aerobics for elderly
    - **Flexibility:** maintain or increase joint flexibility
    Examples: slow stretching exercises; have patient hold stretch 20

seconds and release, then rehold 20 seconds, attempting to reach a little farther
- **Posture:** emphasize potential problem areas—forward head, rounded shoulders, and tight hip flexor muscles
  Examples: teach chin tucks, pectoral stretch, and hip extension stretch
- **Balance coordination:** improve balance and coordination to assist with safety
  Examples: yoga exercises, balance exercises such as standing on one foot, walking a line, and moving objects from one place to another
- **Gait:** teach gait with an assitive device
  Examples: teaching patient the correct side to hold a cane and which lower extremity to advance first
- **Home safety:** teach patient how to perform a safety home assessment
  Examples: provide patient with a safety checklist form to take home and inventory list for safety issues (sample question: are there any throw rugs on the floor?)

18. Education of patient/family and support system
    - Increase ability to perform activities of daily living
    - Home education
    - Patient education brochures and videos
    - Safety education
    - Nutrition counseling
    - Referral to other services as necessary

Chapter Eighteen
Sample Test Questions

1. *You are evaluating a 26-year-old male patient status post arthro-scopic surgery. The physician requests that you evaluate the muscles that insert into the pes anserinus. You have the patient flex the knee and medially rotate the leg while the knee is flexed. Of the muscles listed below, which are you not evaluating?*
    - A. Gracilis
    - B. Sartorius
    - C. Semimembranosus
    - D. Semitendinosus

2. *You are treating a patient secondary to a foot injury. The patient reports that his podiatrist thought the spring ligament was injured as a result of his fall. Which of the following best describes the spring ligament of the foot?*
    - A. It is also called the plantar calcaneocuboid ligament
    - B. It is called the short plantar ligament
    - C. It helps to maintain the medial arch of the foot by supporting the head of the talipes
    - D. The spring ligament is not highly elastic

3. *A patient who has a lesion of the inferior gluteal nerve is referred to the clinic. Which of the following motions would most likely be affected to the greatest extent secondary to an inferior gluteal nerve lesion?*
    - A. Hip abduction
    - B. Hip adduction
    - C. Hip flexion
    - D. Hip extension

4. *The physician has sent a patient to the clinic for a brace that will assist in controlling knee rotation and adduction. Which of the following ligaments was most likely injured?*
    A. Anterior cruciate ligament
    B. Posterior cruciate ligament
    C. Medial collateral ligament
    D. Lateral collateral ligament

5. *When performing ultrasound on a patient it is important to be aware of contraindications for its utilization. One contraindication is performing ultrasound over the epiphyseal or growth plate of a child. Which of the following statements is not true concerning the growth plate?*
    A. It serves as a site of progressive lengthening that is needed in the long bones
    B. It lies between the epiphysis and diaphysis as a transverse disc
    C. It is formed of cartilage
    D. It is found in all bones

6. *Bursae may be found in most of the locations within the body. In which of the following anatomical areas would the bursae most likely not be found?*
    A. Subtendinous
    B. Intramuscular
    C. Subcutaneous
    D. Subfacial

7. *In a class on clinical pathology, the professor asks you what lupus erythematous, scleroderma and dermatomycosis have in common. They can best be grouped together as which of the following?*
    A. Acute infections
    B. Acute bacterial diseases
    C. Collagen vascular diseases
    D. Circulatory disorders

8. In clinical pathology class, the professor describes a pathological disease that involves the arteries and veins of the lower extremity. The symptoms are inflammation, venous thrombosis, and ischemia of the feet. Which of the following diseases is being described by the professor?

A. Raynaud's disease
B. Thromboangiitis obliterans
C. Thrombophlebitis
D. Pitting edema

9. You are treating a patient who is complaining of right shoulder pain. The patient has been diagnosed with a frozen adhesive capsulated shoulder. Which of the following would describe the capsular pattern of the glenohumeral joint?

A. External rotation, abduction, internal rotation
B. External rotation, internal rotation, abduction
C. Internal rotation, abduction, external rotation
D. Abduction, external rotation, internal rotation

10. A patient is sent to physical therapy secondary to a lower extremity injury. Reading the patient's past medical history, you note that the superficial peroneal nerve has been severed. Which of the following muscles would be emphasized in your treatment program?

A. Tibialis anterior
B. Peroneus tertius
C. Peroneus brevis
D. Extensor hallucis longus

11. You are in cardiology class studying the difference between cardiac muscle versus skeletal muscle. It is known that the cardiac muscle is physiologically different from skeletal muscle. Which of the following statements best describes this?

A. It has no bony attachments
B. The actin and myosin filaments produce a different type of striation
C. It does not develop a length-tension relationship
D. It divides into atrial and ventricular proportions

12. *While studying cardiology you are learning about cardiac output.*
    Cardiac output refers to the amount of blood pumped by the heart
    in a specific time period. Which of the following best describes
    cardiac output?
    A. Blood pumped by the heart in a 24-hour period
    B. Blood pumped by the heart in 1 hour
    C. Blood pumped by the heart during a 60-second period
    D. Blood pumped by the heart during an 8-hour period

13. *You are working with a patient who has a small stroke volume and*
    pulse pressure. Which of the following lesions does the patient
    most likely have?
    A. Atrial sclerotic disease
    B. Mitral stenosis
    C. Congestive heart failure
    D. Myocardial infarct

14. *Which of the following is the most frequent location for a myocar-*
    dial infarction to occur?
    A. Left atrium
    B. Left ventricle
    C. Right atrium
    D. Right ventricle

15. *Which of the following is the most common cause of a CVA (cere-*
    brovascular accident) in older adults?
    A. Aneurysm
    B. Hemorrhaging
    C. High blood pressure
    D. Thrombosis

16. *Which of the following actions of the drug Digitalis is common in*
    a patient with chronic congestive heart failure?
    A. A decrease in heart rate
    B. An increase in heart rate
    C. A decrease in the strength of the contraction
    D. No effect on heart rate

17. *You are a physical therapist at the site of a football game as a medical staff member. You watch one of the players fall from a blow to the head and determine by a field evaluation that he has suffered a concussion. Which of the following best defines a concussion?*
    A. Any severe blow to the head
    B. A fracture of the skull
    C. Swelling of the brain as a result of trauma
    D. A temporary state of paralysis of the nervous function, including loss of consciousness

18. *Rheumatoid arthritis can cause many symptoms in its later stages. Which of the following symptoms would most likely be common in a patient who has had rheumatoid arthritis for a long period of time?*
    A. Radial deviation of the fingers
    B. Enlargement of Heberden's nodes
    C. Ulnar deviation of the fingers
    D. Increased muscle strength

19. *You are studying the various types of arthritis, specifically rheumatoid arthritis versus osteoarthritis. Which of the following would best describe the etiology of osteoarthritis?*
    A. Trauma to a joint recently
    B. Under weight
    C. Degeneration caused by aging
    D. Recent injury to the joint

20. *Which of the following definitions best describes the anatomical dead space?*
    A. The portion of the pulmonary tree that is inelastic and does not change size with inspiration or expiration
    B. An area occupied in the airways that does not permit gas exchange
    C. The pulmonary area with the least blood supply
    D. The portion of the pulmonary tree that is not supplied with sensory nerves

21. *You are in physiology class studying tissue excitation. In regard to the strength/duration curve, which of the following is not a true statement?*
    A. It may be considered valuable in testing for nerve degeneration
    B. It may be considered valuable in testing for nerve regeneration
    C. It shows the relationship of current intensity to the duration of reaching expectation threshold
    D. It exhibits development and fatigue during a prolonged stimulus

22. *In a class on physiology of exercise, you are studying the energy needed for muscle contractions. Which of the following statements is false in regard to energy for muscle contractions?*
    A. Energy is produced during aerobic metabolism
    B. Energy is produced during anaerobic metabolism
    C. Energy may be stored as creatine phosphate
    D. Energy is derived from ATP (adenosine triphosphate)

23. *You are studying diabetes mellitus and diabetes insipidus in your clinical pathology course. Which of the following statements is not true about diabetes mellitus, but best describes diabetes insipidus?*
    A. It is a disorder of carbohydrate metabolism
    B. It results from insulin deficiency
    C. It is associated with the pancrease
    D. It is associated with the pituitary gland

24. *Which of the following gestational timeframes is the most susceptible for injury to the fetal cardiovascular system? It is during this timeframe that the fetal cardiovascular system produces most congenital defects.*
    A. Third month
    B. Sixth month
    C. Between the 21st and 40th days
    D. Conception and the 20th day

25. *A patient comes to the clinic with an injury to the skin as a result of exposure to excessive heat. Which of the following listed below will be the first response to this type of skin injury?*
   A. The fluids will seep into the damaged tissue
   B. The blood vessels will become dilated and more permeable secondary to inflammation
   C. Phagocytic cells will remove dead cells and debridement of the area will occur
   D. Blood clotting will occur

26. *The professor is presenting a lecture on the advantages and disadvantages of the following exercises: Isometric, isokinetic, isotonic, and eccentric contractions. The professor informs the class that some of the disadvantages of a particular exercise are that it loads muscle at the weakest point and the momentum factor in lifting. These disadvantages best describe which of the following classifications of exercise?*
   A. Isometric
   B. Isotonic
   C. Isokinetic
   D. Free weights

27. *The patient has experienced a lesion in the frontal lobe of the cerebral hemisphere. Which of the following would most likely be affected?*
   A. Vision
   B. Sensory perception and interpretation
   C. Personality and speech
   D. Hearing and comprehension of speech

28. *A patient experiences an injury resulting in a lesion of the occipital lobe of the cerebral hemisphere. Which of the following are most likely involved?*
   A. Vision and interpretation of visual data
   B. Sensory perception and interpretation
   C. Intelligence and personality
   D. Comprehension of speech and memory

29. *An 18-year-old male tests positive for shoulder dislocation. This patient may have complications as a result of this shoulder dislocation. Which of the following would most likely be involved if the patient were to have complications?*
    A. Axillary artery
    B. Axillary nerve
    C. Radial artery
    D. Radial nerve

30. *In studying physical therapy you are learning about the differences between various spina bifida disorders. You are specifically studying spina bifida myelocele. Which of the following would best describe this disorder?*
    A. A soft tissue tumor in the meninges
    B. A soft tissue tumor in the spinal cord
    C. The most severe form of spina bifida
    D. A herniated sac contained within the spinal cord

31. *A patient reports to physical therapy with a diagnosis of a lesion in the lateral cord of the brachial plexus. Which of the following would you most likely detect upon treatment of this patient?*
    A. Paralysis of the biceps, coracobrachialis, and finger flexors
    B. Paralysis of the deltoid
    C. Paralysis of wrist extension
    D. Paralysis of the hand

32. *You are performing physical therapy on a patient status post cerebrovascular accident. The patient is having difficulty with trunk control and transfers from supine to sit and left to right sidelying. In performing PNF techniques on this patient, which of the following would be best to utilize to assist this patient?*
    A. Hold and relax
    B. Rhythmic initiation
    C. Rhythmic stabilization
    D. Slow reversal hold

33. *In studying the pulmonary system of a patient, you are discussing site of gas exchange in the pulmonary system. Which of the following is the most likely site of gas exchange?*
    A. Alveoli
    B. Bronchi
    C. Brachialis
    D. Trachea

34. *You are performing passive range of motion on a pulmonary patient. What effect will passive range of motion have on this patient's pulmonary ventilation?*
    A. No effect
    B. An undetermined effect
    C. A response proportional to the number of joints involved in passive range of motion
    D. A response proportional to the speed and duration of exercises administered

35. *You have a patient who has episodes of dyspnea and difficulty in expiration. Which of the following would your patient most likely be experiencing?*
    A. Asthma
    B. Bronchitis
    C. Emphysema
    D. Cystic fibrosis

36. *The client has been positioned on his side. You would anticipate that which of the following areas would be a pressure point in this position?*
    A. Sacrum
    B. Occiput
    C. Ankles
    D. Heels

37. *The patient is a 26-year-old male, status post ankle fracture. The physician orders mobilization to increase joint range of motion. Which of the following is the maximum loose-packed position of the ankle joint?*

A. 10° plantar flexion
B. 5° plantar flexion
C. 0° plantar flexion
D. 15° plantar flexion

38. *You are treating a patient status post total hip replacement. You notice in the patient's chart that the patient has received a cemented total hip replacement. Which of the following is not an advantage of a cemented hip?*
    A. It allows early weightbearing
    B. Surgeons report a 90% success rate
    C. There is less postoperative pain
    D. It requires less bone tissue removal

39. *In class you are studying the elbow joint and optimum force output. Which of the following would be the position for elbow flexion in terms of the greatest advantage of optimum force output?*
    A. 120° of elbow flexion
    B. Flexion supination
    C. Midposition or semiprone
    D. 90° of elbow flexion

40. *In anatomy class you are studying the tendinous cuff muscles, also called SITS (supraspinatus, infraspinatus, teres minor). Which of the following does the combined action of the tendinous cuff muscles produce?*
    A. Abduction of the shoulder
    B. External rotation of the shoulder
    C. Pulling of the humerus upward and outward
    D. Depression of the head of the humerus

41. *Your patient is a 26-year-old paraplegic. You are observing the patient standing with braces for a prolonged time. For the paraplegic, prolonged standing with braces in a lordotic position may result in which of the following?*
    A. Stretching of the hip flexors
    B. Stretching of the hip extensors
    C. Stretching of the hip extensors and iliofemoral ligament
    D. Stretching of the ischial femoral ligament

42. *You are in anatomy class studying motions of the wrist. It is known that the motion that the wrist produces is actually a combination of several motions at several different articulations. Which of the following would best describe the axis of motion for the radial and ulnar deviation?*
   A. It lies in the coronal plane through the lunate
   B. It lies in the sagittal plane through the trapezoid
   C. It lies in the sagittal plane through the capitate
   D. It lies in the coronal plane through the capitate

43. *You are performing a test on a patient for hip flexor length. Upon testing the hip, the extremity being tested abducts and remains slightly flexed when lowered to the table. Which of the following would you most likely suspect of muscle tightness?*
   A. Psoas major
   B. Tensor fascia latae
   C. Semitendinosus
   D. Rectus femoris

44. *On the patient described above, you decide to measure normal expansion at the xiphoid process. Which of the following would be the normal value for expansion when measured at the xiphoid process?*
   A. 5 to 10 cm
   B. 5 to 10 in
   C. .5 to 1.0 cm
   D. .5 to 1.0 in

45. *You are performing a postural examination on a 16-year-old track and field star. Upon posture evaluation you notice that the patient has pronated feet. Which of the following would best describe this condition?*
   A. Lateral convexity of the Achilles' tendon due to a medial weight line
   B. Eversion of the calcaneus with lateral convexity of the Achilles' tendon
   C. Eversion of the calcaneus with a medial weight line
   D. Inversion of the calcaneus with a medial weight line

46. *You are in rheumatology class studying degenerative joint disease. The instructor asks you where Heberden's nodes are most frequently located as a result of degenerative joint disease. Which of the following is the correct answer?*
    A. Distal and proximal interphalangeal joints of the fingers
    B. Distal and proximal interphalangeal joints of the fingers and toes
    C. Distal interphalangeal joints of the fingers
    D. Distal interphalangeal joints of the toes

47. *You are performing a gait evaluation on a cross-country track runner who pulled a hamstring muscle. During which period of time in the patient's gait cycle would the hamstring muscle be the most active?*
    A. Midstance to heel-off
    B. Swing phase
    C. Acceleration to midswing
    D. Midswing to deceleration

48. *You are performing palpation on a patient with general lower back pain. Which of the following landmarks would be most helpful to isolate the L4 vertebral level upon palpation of this patient?*
    A. Anterior superior iliac spine
    B. Posterior superior iliac spine
    C. Iliac crest
    D. Greater trochanter

49. *Your patient is a 56-year-old female with a diagnosis of a herniated disc between vertebrae C6 and C7. During a conversation with the physician, he informs you that the patient has a C7 nerve root impingement. Upon testing this patient, you expect weakness in all of the following motor activities except for which one?*
    A. Wrist flexion
    B. Finger flexion
    C. Finger extension
    D. Elbow extension

50. *You are performing ultrasound under water to a patient's left hand. In performing the ultrasound under water, which of the following would be the most important safety factor to be considered?*
   A. Utilizing a plastic bucket instead of a metal whirlpool
   B. Keeping the ultrasound head moving
   C. Keeping the ultrasound watts per centimeters squared under 1.0
   D. Connecting the ultrasound to a ground fault interruption circuit

51. *You have been called into the physical therapy department secondary to a patient being brought into the emergency room with severe burns on both posterior lower extremities. The physician instructs you to begin working with this newly admitted burn patient. Which of the following would be your first priority?*
   A. Performing an evaluation on the wound area
   B. Splinting to control contractures and edema
   C. Closing the wound
   D. Beginning immediate wound cleaning, debridement, and sterile dressing

52. *The physician has instructed you to perform ultrasound under water secondary to a patient experiencing foot pain in the medial arch. When administering ultrasound under water, which of the following would be the best position for the sound head?*
   A. The sound head should be in direct contact with the medial arch of the foot
   B. The sound head should be approximately 3 inches away from the medial arch of the foot
   C. The sound head should be approximately 1 inch away from the medial arch of the foot
   D. The sound head should be approximately 9 cm from the medial arch of the foot

53. *You are a physical therapist who has been instructed by a physician to lead an exercise group of 20 geriatric patients at the community center. The physician suggests that you emphasize areas that typically show reduced range of motion for geriatric patients. Which of the actions listed below would not be an emphasis of your program?*

    A. Hip flexion
    B. Hip extension
    C. Pectoralis muscle stretch
    D. Chin glides, chin tucks

54. *During the swing phase, acceleration stage, which muscles remain active throughout the entire stage to help shorten the extremity so it can clear the ground by holding the ankle in a neutral position?*
    A. Tibialis posterior, peroneus brevis
    B. Tibialis anterior, peroneus tertius
    C. Tibialis anterior, peroneus tertius, extensor hallucis longus
    D. Tibialis posterior, peroneus tertius, extensor hallucis longus

55. *During the swing phase, deceleration stage, which muscles contract to slow down the swing phase just prior to heel strike, thus permitting the heel to strike quietly in a controlled manner?*
    A. Gluteus medius
    B. Gluteus maximus
    C. Hamstring
    D. Quadriceps

56. *Your patient is an 18-year-old male who was seriously injured in a motorcycle accident. The radiology examination reveals a fracture described as one in which the ends are driven into each other. Of the choices listed below, what is the typical name for this type of fracture?*
    A. Comminuted
    B. Impacted
    C. Displaced
    D. Intraarticular

57. *Muscular contraction of the cardiac chambers is different from the electrical conduction system. The normal conduction pathway for muscular contraction of the heart to follow is which of the patterns listed below?*
    A. Left atrium, right atrium, ventricles
    B. Right atrium, left atrium, ventricles
    C. Right ventricle, left ventricle, atrium
    D. Left ventricle, right ventricle, atrium

58. *The sinus node acts as the cardiac pacemaker in the heart. The sinus node is a group of cardiac cells that discharges an impulse. Where is the sinus node located in the heart?*
    A. Right atrium
    B. Left atrium
    C. Right ventricle
    D. Left ventricle

59. *On rounds you observe a 72-year-old male with pectus carinatum, more commonly known as pigeon chest. Which of the following best describes his condition?*
    A. Lower portion of the sternum is depressed
    B. Lateral diameter of the chest is increased
    C. Sternum is displaced anteriorly, increasing anterior-posterior diameter
    D. Sternum is displaced posteriorly, increasing anterior-posterior diameter

60. *A patient enters the clinic with an injury to the brachioradialis muscle of the left forearm. The patient was injured when he was delivering a piano and the lid slammed down on his forearm. The patient now has limited action of the left forearm. With an injury to the brachioradialis muscle, which action/actions would now be limited in this patient?*
    A. Forearm supination
    B. Forearm supination, elbow flexion, wrist flexion
    C. Forearm pronation, elbow flexion
    D. Forearm pronation, supination, elbow flexion

61. *Several muscles in the body have dual innervation, which is innervation by more than one nerve. Which of the following muscles does not have dual innervation?*
    A. Flexor digitorum profundus
    B. Flexor carpi ulnaris
    C. Flexor pollicis brevis
    D. Lumbricales

62. *A 16-year-old soccer player enters the emergency room with an anterior tibialis muscle injury sustained during practice. The patient has significant bruising and discoloration in the area. Which nerve innervates the anterior tibialis muscle and may be tested in this patient?*
    A. Lateral plantar
    B. Superficial peroneal
    C. Tibial
    D. Deep peroneal

63. *In a class on gross anatomy, the professor asks you to dissect the muscles that attach to the ischial tuberosity. Which group of muscles listed below attaches to the ischial tuberosity?*
    A. Biceps femoris, semitendinosus
    B. Semimembranosus, biceps femoris
    C. Semimembranosus, biceps femoris, semitendinosus
    D. Semimembranosus, semitendinosus

64. *During an internship in the neurology unit at a major university hospital, the neurosurgeon asks you to perform the test for reflex C5. Which of the following should be tested to determine the reflex at level C5?*
    A. Elbow extension
    B. Triceps
    C. Biceps
    D. Brachioradialis

65. *A patient enters the clinic with a prescription for direct current electrical stimulation. Upon reading the order you notice that the patient's diagnosis is Bell's palsy. Of the following, which nerve would you determine to be injured in this patient?*
    A. Trigeminal
    B. Trochlear
    C. Facial
    D. Vagus

66. *You are evaluating a patient with a repetitive motion injury from work. You have tested the patient's pronation/supination of the forearm and wrist flexion/extension. Which of the following muscles does not assist in pronation of the radioulnar joint?*
    A. Brachioradialis
    B. Flexor carpi radialis
    C. Pronator quadratus
    D. Flexor carpi ulnaris

67. *A butcher is responsible for processing meat packaging. In the process of carving the meat he injures the second and third digits of his hand. The hand surgeon reports that the nerves in the second and third digits have been permanently injured. Which nerve/nerves would be injured?*
    A. Ulnar nerve
    B. Median nerve
    C. Radial nerve
    D. Ulnar/median

68. *When studying upper motor neuron lesions in neuroanatomy, you determine that which of the following is not a characteristic typically seen with this type of lesion?*
    A. Muscle atrophy
    B. Spasticity
    C. Hyperreflexia
    D. Babinski sign possible

69. *A 26-year-old triathlete has just completed a competitive event in swimming, biking, and running. The patient has extreme muscle fatigue after this event. Which of the following may build up in the body and cause muscle fatigue?*
    A. Glycogen
    B. Lactic acid
    C. Fatty acids
    D. Glucose

70. *In determining a target heart rate for a 62-year-old patient, you would use the calculation for maximum heart rate. Which of the following best describes the calculation for maximum heart rate?*
    A. Pulse rate for 60 seconds
    B. Count pluse for 15 seconds x 4, plus age
    C. (220 plus age)
    D. (220 minus age)

71. *A patient undergoes open heart surgery at a prestigious heart hospital. The patient is being evaluated 1 day postoperative for possible placement in the acute inpatient cardiac rehab program. The patient's blood pressure reading indicates hypertension. Which of the following readings would be considered indicative of hypertension?*
    A. 120/80
    B. Above 120/80
    C. Above 140/90
    D. Under 120/90

72. *A patient comes to you from the hand surgeon with a request to specifically evaluate the anatomical snuffbox. The hand surgeon is concerned that the patient might have suffered an injury to the nerve crossing the anatomical snuffbox. Of the following nerves, which would you need to evaluate?*
    A. Radial
    B. Median
    C. Ulnar
    D. Musculocutaneous

73. *A patient comes to you status post ankle sprain which is healing well. The patient needs to increase range of motion to resume full activity. Of the following, which movement will take place in the ankle subtalar joint?*
    A. Pronation/supination
    B. Eversion/inversion
    C. Adduction/abduction
    D. Dorsiflexion

74. *An 8-year-old male enters the clinic with a diagnosis of fracture of the distal radius. The patient's mother reports that the patient was riding his bicycle down a steep hill when he fell off. The physician sends the patient to you for evaluation because he is concerned about possible nerve damage. A fracture of the distal radius will result in possible nerve damage to which nerve?*
   A. Musculocutaneous
   B. Radial
   C. Ulnar
   D. Median

75. *A patient comes to the clinic with a swollen right thumb. He reports that he was at work operating a press machine when the press closed and caught his thumb. The patient will need joint immobilization to restore range of motion; otherwise he has escaped with minimal injury. The carpometacarpal joint of the thumb is classified as what type of joint?*
   A. Uniaxial
   B. Biaxial
   C. Saddle
   D. Hinge

76. *A muscle is known to have a proximal and distal attachment. It is necessary to know the attachments for palpation and manual muscle tests. Which of the following is the proximal attachment of a limb muscle?*
   A. Tendon
   B. Insertion
   C. Belly of muscle
   D. Origin

77. *A patient enters the clinic with what appears to be pinched nerves in the cervical spine area. The patient is reporting radiating symptoms into the left upper extremity that follow no particular dermatome pattern. The patient reports that he is going to have a test in which some type of electrodes are inserted into the muscle to test which nerves are injured. Based on this information, which of the following tests is the patient most likely having?*

A. Electromyogram
B. Arthroscopy
C. EKG
D. Myelogram

78. *Your neuroanatomy professor lectures on the divisions of the brain. The brain is divided into three major divisions. Which of the following is not one of the three major brain regions?*
    A. Brainstem
    B. Midbrain
    C. Cerebellum
    D. Cerebrum

79. *A pregnant patient is advised to avoid the Valsalva maneuver during her pregnancy. What effect listed below does the Valsalva maneuver have?*
    A. Increase in intrathoracic pressure
    B. Decrease in intrathoracic pressure
    C. Pressure remains the same, no effect
    D. Increase in inspiration needs

80. *You are in physiology class studying the difference between erythrocytes and leukocytes in the body. Each one has a primary function to perform so that the body functions normally. Which of the following would be a primary function of erythrocytes in the body?*
    A. Transport oxygen
    B. Carry iron
    C. Produce calcium
    D. Produce red blood cells

81. *You are continuing your studies in neurology on abnormal reflexes. You are now focusing on the reflex called the flexor withdrawal. The flexor withdrawal integration level is spinal. Where would the stimulus be applied to test the flexor withdrawal?*
    A. Sole of the foot with lower extremity in extension
    B. Sole of the foot with lower extremity in flexion
    C. Forefoot with the lower extremity in extension
    D. Forefoot with the lower extremity in flexion

82. *You are testing the tonic labyrinthine reflex of a patient. You have positioned the patient supine. Which of the following would you consider to be a positive response to this position?*
    A. Increased extensor tone
    B. Increased flexor tone
    C. Increased extensor tone in upper extremities and flexor tone
    D. Increased flexor tone in upper extremities and extensor tone in lower extremities

83. *You are testing a patient for the negative support reaction. The integration level for the negative support reaction is the brainstem. You bounce the patient several times on the soles of the feet but you do not allow her to bear weight. Which of the following would you anticipate as the patient's response?*
    A. Increased extensor tone in lower extremities
    B. Increased extensor tone in upper extremities
    C. Increased flexor tone in lower extremities
    D. Increased extensor tone in upper extremities

84. *You have a patient referred to physical therapy with cerebral palsy. Which of the following does not describe what you would typically observe in a cerebral palsy child?*
    A. The child may be either passive or stiff
    B. The child cannot adjust the body position
    C. The child can hold or bring the head into a normal position
    D. The child may be classified as either spastic or ataxic

85. *A physician informs you that he feels that the patient is pretending to be ill to arouse sympathy for his condition. He suspects that the patient is slow to recuperate because he continues to receive benefits from the insurance company during a slow recovery. Which of the following most likely describes this individual?*
    A. Patient is negligent
    B. Patient is a hypochondriac
    C. Patient is a malinger
    D. Patient is paranoid

86. *A patient comes to physical therapy for further instructions on crutch ambulation. Upon observation you notice that the patient moves the left crutch first, then the right leg, then the right crutch, then the left leg. Of the following, which type of crutch gait have you most likely observed?*
    A. Three-point gait
    B. Two-point gait
    C. Swing-through
    D. Four-point gait

87. *A patient is referred to physical therapy several months status post hip burn. The patient reports that he had an allograft over the burn area. Which of the following does this describe?*
    A. The graft skin is from the same species
    B. The graft skin is from the same individual
    C. The graft skin is from an animal
    D. A surgical incision in the form of the letter Z, the length of the graft

88. *You are performing a musculoskeletal examination of a patient's thoracic lumbar spine. Which of the tests listed below would best determine if there is an impingement of the nerve in the thoracic lumbar root level?*
    A. Compression test
    B. Distraction test
    C. Ely's test
    D. Slump test

89. *You are performing a neurological evaluation on a patient that has had a vascular injury. The patient has the following impairment: loss of consciousness, coma, no ability to speak, and hemiplegia. Based on this information, in which of the following areas does this vascular involvement occur?*
    A. Anterior cerebral artery
    B. Middle cerebral artery
    C. Posterior cerebral artery
    D. Vertebrobasilar artery

90. *According to the American Physical Therapy Association* Standards of Care, *the initial evaluation should include all of the following except?*
    A. Diagnosis
    B. Social environment needs
    C. Functional status
    D. Medication

91. *You are evaluating a patient with a diagnosis of Marie-Strumpell disease. The physician instructs you to evaluate the patient and determine an appropriate treatment program. Which of the following would be the best treatment program for this patient?*
    A. Rest and medication
    B. Joint mobility, heat, and postural instructions
    C. Aspirin in high dosages
    D. Resistive exercises and stretching

92. *You are instructed to perform vascular testing on a 35-year-old female with peripheral vascular disease. The physician sends this patient to your department for evaluation and set-up of an appropriate treatment program. Which of the following tests would be the least important in evaluating this patient's condition?*
    A. Rubor test
    B. Girth measurements
    C. Volumetric measurement
    D. Deep pressure test

93. *You are performing an upper extremity evaluation on a patient with an injury to the right shoulder. You are evaluating the muscles that attach to the greater tuberosity of the humerus. In planning this patient's treatment program, which of the following muscles would not be emphasized?*
    A. Supraspinatus
    B. Infraspinatus
    C. Teres minor
    D. Subscapularis

94. *You have a 42-year-old female status post removal of the lymphatic system in the axillary region secondary to cancer. The physician wants you to work on edema through measurement for a pressure garment and massage 1-day post surgery. How should the massage be performed for best results?*
    A. You decide not to do massage but Jobst compression pump
    B. Massage the proximal segment first
    C. Massage the distal segment first
    D. Order a garment and check on the patient daily

95. *A patient postoperative removal of the lymphatic system in the axillary region is very concerned about the cancer spreading. You read in her chart that the physician was not able to remove all of the cancer; it has spread. At the next treatment session she asks you if the surgery was successful. Since the physician is inaccessible, what do you tell her?*
    A. You are deeply sorry, but it was not 100% successful
    B. You are deeply sorry, but you are sure the doctor did the best he could, as he is one of the top surgeons
    C. You have no idea whether or not surgery was successful
    D. Tell her you are not able to provide that information; she will have to discuss it with her surgeon

96. *You have a 26-year-old female 2 days post hand laceration. The doctor orders paraffin treatments and range of motion. What should be the typical treatment temperature for paraffin?*
    A. 50°C
    B. 30°C
    C. 40°C
    D. 126°C

97. *You are working at a hospital that has not approved the SOAP note format, but instead uses the problem-oriented medical record format. What are the four major components of the POMR format?*
    A. Subjective, objective, assessment, plan
    B. Subjective, objective, progress, potential for rehabilitation
    C. Subjective, laboratory test with physician medical history, assessment, prognosis for rehabilitation
    D. Subjective, treatment plan, assessment, prognosis

98. *In the hospital where you work, the policy states all notes must be written in the SOAP format. Your patient tells you that his chief concern is limited movement or loss of range of motion in the left shoulder. Where does this information go in the SOAP format?*
    A. Subjective
    B. Objective
    C. Assessment
    D. Plan

99. *This disorder affects bone formation and is transmitted as an autosomal dominant factor. The result is the long bones of the limbs remain short. What is the medical name for this condition?*
    A. Osteogenesis imperfecta
    B. Bone tumor
    C. Achondroplasia
    D. Fibrous dysplasia

100. *The chart review reveals a patient with a condition known as thyrotoxicosis. This condition is due to hyperthyroidism. The disease is characterized by an enlargement of the thyroid gland. What is not another more common name for this disease?*
    A. Grave's disease
    B. Primary hyperthyroidism
    C. Secondary hyperthyroidism
    D. Fibrous dysplasia

101. *You are given the description of a type of electrical stimulation as follows: medium-frequency current, approximately 4000 Hz, and four electrodes in a crossed pattern on the patient. What type of electrical stimulation is most likely being described?*
    A. Low-volt electric stimulation
    B. High-volt electric stimulation
    C. Russian stimulation
    D. Interferential current stimulation

102. *There is a special type of electrical stimulation whose primary purpose is to alleviate pain for a patient. There are minimal side effects and the patient can utilize this unit 24 hours a day. What is the name for this type of electrical stimulation?*

A. Transcutaneous electrical nerve stimulation
B. High-volt stimulation
C. Low-volt stimulation
D. Russian stimulation

103. *The hip musculature involves several muscle groups for different actions. Hip abduction takes place with nerve innervation from the superior gluteal nerve. Which muscles compose the hip abductor group?*
   A. Psoas major, iliacus, sartorius
   B. Gluteus medius, gluteus minimus, tensor fasciae latae
   C. Gluteus medius, gluteus minimus, sartorius
   D. Gluteus medius, gracilis, pectineus

104. *The patient injured the hip adductor muscles in a track race while jumping hurdles. The patient comes to the clinic with pain in the hip adductor muscle group. Several nerves innervate the hip adductor muscle group. Which nerves innervate the hip adductor muscles?*
   A. Femoral, tibial
   B. Femoral, superior gluteal
   C. Femoral, obturator, tibial
   D. Femoral, obturator, inferior gluteal

105. *A 21-year-old female sprains her ankle at a basketball game. You are the medical staff member attending the game. You notice that swelling is beginning but she insists on continuing to play. Which of the following modalities would not decrease swelling?*
   A. Ice massage
   B. Cryopressure
   C. Ice towel
   D. Evaporative coolants

106. *A patient with inflammation comes to the clinic with evaluation and treatment orders. Which of the following modalities could be utilized to place chemical substances into the body with direct current to decrease inflammation?*
   A. Myoflex with ultrasound
   B. Phonophoresis
   C. Iontophoresis
   D. Ultrasound

107. *You are working with a physical therapist student when performing short-wave diathermy on a 36-year-old female patient. You explain that this treatment is an example of heat transferred by energy. Which term listed below correctly identifies this type of heat transfer?*
    A. Conversion
    B. Convection
    C. Conduction
    D. Radiation

108. *In physical therapy you may utilize physical or mechanical techniques, as well as manual therapy techniques. Which of the following is not an example of manual therapy techniques performed by a physical therapist?*
    A. Grade-one mobilization
    B. Grade-two mobilization
    C. Grade-three mobilization
    D. Grade-five mobilization

109. *You have a patient reporting neck pain with a bulging disc at level C6-C7. During the history, the patient tells you that she also suffers from TMJ problems. The physician's order is for cervical traction. What would be best for this patient?*
    A. Do not perform cervical traction secondary to medical history
    B. Sitting cervical traction
    C. Supine cervical traction with cervical spine pillow
    D. Saunders cervical traction device

110. *Your patient is a 44-year-old female with low back pain resulting from no apparent cause/reason. You decide to set her up in traction with a hold period of 40 seconds, rest period 10 seconds, for 20 minutes at 60 pounds. What type of traction does this best describe?*
    A. Autotraction
    B. Gravity lumbar traction
    C. Manual traction
    D. Intermittent mechanical traction

111. *Psychology of a patient can play an important part in his or her physical therapy. Physical therapists may treat patients who are in the psychiatric ward of a hospital for a wide range of musculoskeletal conditions. The chart of a psych patient you are treating provides the following information: patient exhibits psychotic behavior, suspicious, resentful and rigid. What does this description most likely describe?*
    A. Hypochondria
    B. Hysteria
    C. Paranoia
    D. Depression

112. *You are on rounds in the psychiatric ward as a physical therapist intern. You are given the following information on a patient: he is pessimistic, irritable, lacks self-confidence, and has a gloomy outlook on life. What would be the most likely diagnosis, or problem, this patient is experiencing?*
    A. Hysteria
    B. Depression
    C. Psychopathy
    D. Schizophrenia

113. *The patient you are working with is a 28-year-old head injury victim of a brutal beating in an alley. The patient clinically demonstrates excessive tone in the limbs, which are resistant to both active and passive movement. Which term listed below would best describe this condition?*
    A. Flaccidity
    B. Hypotonia
    C. Hypertonia
    D. Rigidity

114. *You are teaching a spinal cord injury patient proper pressure relief in the wheelchair. You explain that every 10 to 15 minutes he will need to provide pressure relief independently to prevent sores or ulcers. What is the minimal level of injury this patient can have in order to be able to provide independent care for himself?*
    A. C4
    B. C5
    C. C6
    D. C8

115. *Your last patient of the day is a spinal cord injury patient whom you are teaching self range of motion. You explain that this will be a very important component in the home program. What is the minimal level of injury this patient can have to perform self range of motion independently?*

    A. C7
    B. C8
    C. C5
    D. C4

116. *A 26-year-old female is injured in a motor vehicle accident. The injury results in an incomplete spinal cord lesion. The symptoms are paralysis and loss of sensation, except in the sacral area. What is the correct term for this injury?*

    A. Cauda equina injury
    B. Sacral sparing
    C. Central cord syndrome
    D. Brown-Sequard syndrome

117. *A 12-year-old male is presented to the clinic with hip flexion contractures. The contractures are secondary to fibrosis where the skin is bound down to the tissue. The physician states that the patient has chronic inflammation of the connective tissue. What is the name of this medical condition?*

    A. Chronic contractures
    B. Scleroderma
    C. Fibrositis
    D. Myositis

118. *You are to perform a postural evaluation of a patient from the side or lateral view. Specifically determining normal alignment for the head, scapula, and shoulder, which of the following is normal alignment?*

    A. Head neutral, scapula depressed, shoulder neutral
    B. Head forward, scapula flat, shoulder neutral
    C. Head neutral, scapula flat, shoulder neutral
    D. Head hyperextended, scapula winged, shoulder neutral

119. *A spinal cord patient 2 weeks post MVA is referred to physical therapy for evaluation and prognosis for rehabilitation. What muscle grade in the lower extremity is necessary for functional performance by this individual?*
    A. Fair
    B. Fair plus
    C. Poor plus
    D. Good minus

120. *You are to perform a manual muscle test on a 26-year-old hip patient. The patient can perform full range of motion in supine position for hip adduction/abduction. In sidelying, the patient cannot perform hip adduction/abduction. Using this information, what would you determine this patient's muscle grade to be?*
    A. Poor
    B. Trace
    C. Fair
    D. Zero

121. *You are instructed to perform manual muscle testing on a L3-L4 spinal cord patient, who is a 21-year-old male and uncooperative. Which of the following considerations is not important?*
    A. Informing the patient of what you will be doing
    B. Stabilizing the proximal part
    C. Lining up the origin and insertion
    D. Testing bilaterally, starting with the injured side first

122. *You have a 29-year-old male patient who was involved in a chemical burn accident at work the day before. You are instructed to start whirlpool and debridement treatments at 98°F. What would be the correct temperature conversion to Celsius for this patient?*
    A. 36°C
    B. 50°C
    C. 25°C
    D. 30°C

123. *Several types of contractions may take place with an individual muscle or muscle groups. These are classified in kinesiology with specific terms. Of the following, which is referred to as the muscle group whose contraction is considered to be the principal agent in producing a joint motion?*
    A. Antagonist
    B. Concentric
    C. Agonist
    D. Eccentric

124. *Which physics law can be interpreted clinically to mean that the further the infrared light, for example, is moving away from the patient, the greater the decrease in intensity will be?*
    A. Joule's law
    B. Ohm's law
    C. Inverse square law
    D. Cosine law

125. *You are requested to treat a 56-year-old male in the neurointensive care unit. You find the following results on the patient: no voluntary movement, unresponsive to stimulus, no reflexes, and positive Babinski response. Which most likely describes this patient's condition?*
    A. Cerebrovascular accident
    B. Coma
    C. Stupor
    D. Uncooperative patient

126. *A patient is sent to physical therapy with psoriasis, and the physician orders a third-degree erythemal dosage on the patient. The dosage results in intense reddening 3 to 4 hours post exposure for approximately 3 to 4 days. The patient has slight edema with marked peeling and severe itching. What would be the appropriate treatment frequency for this patient?*
    A. Once a week
    B. Two times a week
    C. Three times a week
    D. Daily

127. *You are an educational instructor of a physical therapist program. You explain to the class that scores on testing are going to be compared to standard deviation of the mean. What percentage of students taking your examination would you expect to score within plus and minus one standard deviation of the mean?*
    A. 68%
    B. 70%
    C. 72%
    D. 50%

128. *It is important to be ethical when performing a research study. Which of the following should take place first for a study to be ethical?*
    A. The patient should be informed that he or she has the right to terminate the experiment at any time
    B. The patient should be debriefed following the experiment
    C. The end results of the experiment should be explained to the patient
    D. The patient should sign the informed consent document

129. *In implementing a treatment program for a patient after a non-surgical ACL reconstruction, which of the following would be the most appropriate exercise to initiate in the beginning stages of rehabilitation?*
    A. Full-range isokinetics for knee flexion and extension
    B. Straight leg raises times six repetitions with maximal weight
    C. Stair machine
    D. N-K table full range of motion times six repetitions with maximal weight

130. *You are a physical therapist providing medical coverage for a high school football game. During the course of the game, one of the football players is knocked down on the field. You rush out to his side and determine that the player is unconscious. What is the first thing you should do in examining the unconscious athlete?*

A. Check breathing and, if breathing is impaired, clear the airway and proceed to give mouth-to-mouth resuscitation if necessary

B. Start with the head and determine first if there is any bleeding or fluid coming from the nose, ears, eyes, or mouth

C. Check for shock

D. Since the victim is unconscious have someone call 911, then proceed to check the airway, breathing, and pulse

131. *You have received a physician's order to discharge an inpatient that has been under your care for a total knee replacement. Which of the following personnel would you contact first to start planning discharge from the hospital to home? Select the most appropriate answer.*

A. The physician

B. Social worker

C. Patient's family

D. Home health agency

132. *You are participating in a track and field event on a hot summer day in July. The temperature is extremely hot with high humidity. The physical therapist that is participating with you becomes severely dehydrated and, with exposure to the severe heat, goes into shock. Your colleague falls to the ground and needs immediate attention. Which of the following is the first step that should be taken?*

A. First check for any wounds to see if bleeding is present

B. Body temperature should be reduced by placing cold towels or cloths on your colleague

C. Body position should be arranged with the head and the trunk higher than the limbs

D. If available, oxygen should be administered

133. *You are working in the spinal cord unit with a C6 spinal cord injury patient. Your functional outcome for this patient is for him or her to be able to perform independent bed mobility with side rails. In planning the treatment program, which of the following muscles would you most likely emphasize?*

A. Pectoralis major
B. Neck musculature
C. Scapula musculature
D. Biceps muscle

134. *You are treating a patient on the field who has the following clinical features: demonstrates muscle twitching and cramping in the lower calf, spasms in the gastrocnemius muscle, and heavy sweating. Which of the following heat disorders is this patient most likely experiencing?*
   A. Heat cramps
   B. Heat syncope
   C. Heat exhaustion
   D. Heat hyperpyrexia

135. *You are testing a pediatric patient for symmetrical tonic reflex. You provide the test stimulus by flexing the patient's head. Which of the following best describes a positive reaction to this test stimulus?*
   A. The arms will flex and the legs will extend
   B. The arms will extend and the legs will flex
   C. The arms will flex and the legs will flex
   D. The arms will extend and the legs will extend

136. *A patient comes to the clinic with burns on the left anterior arm and left anterior leg. You have scheduled sterile whirlpool debridement and preparation of dressings for this patient. Utilizing the Rule of Nines and assuming this patient is an adult, what would be the specific value for the percentage of burns suffered by this patient?*
   A. 4.5%
   B. 9%
   C. 13.5%
   D. 18%

137. *The patient is sent to you for bracing as a result of a fracture at the level of T10 to L1. The physician recommends a rigid high-back brace for stabilization. Which of the following braces would be most appropriate to plan for this patient?*

A. Lumbar corset
B. Taylor brace
C. Knight-Taylor spinal brace
D. Jewett brace

138. *You are working in the physical therapy department with a child who has suffered burns on the left arm and left leg. Utilizing the Rule of Nines, which of the following specific values would correctly describe the percentage of the body burned?*
A. 13.5%
B. 23%
C. 18%
D. 36%

139. *You are treating a patient for arthritis and is reporting wrist pain. You order a typical brace utilized with arthritic patients, which supports the hand in a functional position. Which of the following braces have you ordered for the implementation of the treatment program for this patient?*
A. A wrist cock-up splint
B. A resting hand splint
C. A wrist splint static
D. An ulnar/radial gutter

140. *A patient is seen in physical therapy with a brachial plexus injury. The physician has ordered that a brace or splint be used to protect the patient and promote healing. Which of the following would be correct to implement in the treatment program of a brachial plexus injury?*
A. A shoulder sling
B. A shoulder splint
C. No bracing should be utilized and active motion should be encouraged
D. The patient does not need a shoulder splint but should be given an elbow splint

141. *You are analyzing the gait of an individual with a prosthetic. In evaluating the gait, you notice that the socket has a poor fit and appears to have a weak suspension system, and the knee friction is too soft. Which of the following would be the most likely gait deviation that you would observe?*
    A. Lateral whip
    B. Rotation of the foot at heel strike
    C. Instability of the knee
    D. Pistoning of the socket

142. *You are performing a gait evaluation on a patient who has injured his right lower extremity. In evaluating the patient's gait, you notice that he will not bear weight on the injured extremity. When ambulating he takes a short step to transfer weight to the uninjured side as quickly as possible. Which of the following types of gait would best describe this patient's symptoms?*
    A. Steppage gait
    B. Foot slap
    C. Antalgic gait
    D. Abducted lurch

143. *You are providing an education program to an industry where repetitive motion injuries are commonly seen. To assist in decreasing repetitive injuries within this company, which of the following would be the most important concept to emphasize first?*
    A. Instruct the employees in proper warm-up procedures
    B. Instruct the employees in strengthening exercises
    C. Provide the company with isokinetic testing and the results on each employee
    D. Provide posters on proper body mechanics

144. *A patient is sent to physical therapy with a burn on the posterior aspect of the elbow. The patient has a low pain tolerance and was admitted to the hospital in the early morning. It is afternoon and the patient is sent down for physical therapy. Which of the following would be the most appropriate treatment program?*

A. Active range of motion emphasizing flexion
B. Active range of motion emphasizing extension
C. Passive range of motion emphasizing extension and positioning of the elbow in full extension
D. Whirlpool

145. *In implementing another cardiopulmonary-pulmonary program for a chest physical therapy patient, which of the following positions is most appropriate for the right middle lobe?*
   A. Patient is sitting in the chair leaning forward approximately 20° to 30°, resting on pillows
   B. Patient is in prone position, rotated one-half turn upward, with the bed elevated 18 inches and chest tilted 20°
   C. Patient is prone with pillows under the stomach
   D. Patient is in left sidelying position rotated backward one-half turn, with the bed elevated 14 inches

146. *You are treating an inpatient at a local hospital status post left CVA. The patient is to return home in approximately 2 weeks and you are working on transfers into and out of a vehicle. Which of the following would be the most important to implement in this patient's treatment program?*
   A. Notify the patient's family that the patient will be leaving the hospital in 2 weeks. Request that they come in to learn how to perform transfers into and out of a vehicle.
   B. You have a modified vehicle within the rehabilitation program. Have the patient practice transfers into and out of that vehicle.
   C. Instruct the patient that he or she will be returning home in 2 weeks so it is extremely important to concentrate on transfer techniques and cooperate 100% with you.
   D. Obtain a handicapped parking permit for this patient.

147. *When evaluating a stage-three decubitus ulcer of a patient, which of the following would be the least important to note in the progress notes?*
   A. The size of the wound
   B. Temperature
   C. Hip muscle strength
   D. Drainage and color

148. *You are implementing an exercise program for a patient who is rehabilitated after right shoulder pain. Which of the following would you implement in a treatment program to assist in instructing him or her in functional training and carryover?*
   A. Isokinetic rehabilitation
   B. PNF movements
   C. The shoulder wheel
   D. Dressing and undressing activities

149. *You are analyzing a patient's cardiopulmonary status in the physical therapy department. You notice during chest physical therapy that percussions sound dull with wheezing and crackles upon auscultation. These clinical signs are most likely associated with which one of the following lung pathologies?*
   A. Atelectasis
   B. Pulmonary edema
   C. Pneumonia
   D. Pneumothorax

150. *You have a cardiac patient 3 days postoperative referred to cardiac rehab program. The physician refers the patient to physical therapy for you to implement a treatment program. Which of the following treatment programs would be appropriate for this patient?*
   A. Ambulating 200 yards in a 5-minute period with no EKG changes or changes in symptoms
   B. Lower extremity ergometry x 15 minutes
   C. Lower extremity ergometry x 30 minutes
   D. Upper extremity ergometry x 15 minutes

151. *You are performing a treatment program for a neurological patient. You move the patient's extremity through a predetermined range of motion. This motion is shoulder flexion and extension. Then the patient is requested to repeat the movement on her own. Which of the following are you most likely performing on this patient?*
   A. Kinesthesia
   B. Proprioception
   C. Graphesthesia
   D. Barognosis

152. *A 25-year-old female 6 days post cesarean delivery has been referred to you for training in proper posture and body mechanics. Which of the following would be the proper instructions for body mechanics for a post cesarean patient?*
    A. Whenever sitting, the patient should avoid hard chairs because they have poor back support
    B. When standing, the patient should relax the abdominal muscles in order not to place any strain upon them
    C. When bending over, the patient should keep a flattened lordotic curve in the low back with a wide base of support and legs parallel
    D. When getting up from a lying-down position, the patient should roll over to the side, swinging the legs over the edge and getting up slowly

153. *You are treating a patient who comes to physical therapy complaining of lower thoracic pain. Upon palpation you notice no significant structural or muscular problems. You decide to test the patient's reflexes, particularly the upper abdominal reflex. Which of the following levels are you testing?*
    A. Thoracic 10, 11, 12
    B. Thoracic 8, 9, 10
    C. Thoracic 5, 6, 7
    D. Thoracic 9, 10, 11

154. *A truck driver is sent to physical therapy with a diagnosis of Bell's Palsy. The patient relates that he had been driving for 3 days continuously for periods of 12 to 14 hours on the road. The patient reports that he kept his window rolled down so that he could get fresh air to keep himself awake. What type of treatment program listed below would be most effective for this patient?*
    A. Direct current electrical stimulation to the motor points
    B. Iontophoresis for the inflammation
    C. High-volt electrical stimulation
    D. Massage

155. *The physical therapist is performing an inservice on proper body mechanics to a group of physical therapist assistants. Which of the following best describes the domain in education that deals with motor skills?*
    A. Cognitive
    B. Affective
    C. Psychomotor
    D. Motor skills

156. *You are treating a pediatric patient with cystic fibrosis. The patient suffers from excessive secretions. The physician diagnosed the patient with cystic fibrosis through a sweat test. Which of the following would you implement for an appropriate treatment program for this patient?*
    A. Breathing exercises
    B. Breathing exercises and postural drainage
    C. The physician should order medication therapy
    D. Chest physical therapy

157. *In treating a 36-year-old patient for hip pain you notice, when measuring range of motion, that the patient demonstrates a capsular pattern in the hip. Which of the following best describes the capsular pattern that this patient most likely demonstrates secondary to inflammatory process of the hip?*
    A. Extension, abduction, internal rotation
    B. Flexion, abduction, internal rotation
    C. Flexion, adduction, internal rotation
    D. Internal rotation, flexion, abduction

158. *You are implementing a treatment program for a patient emphasizing equilibrium coordination. Which of the following tests would be important to evaluate equilibrium coordination?*
    A. Observe the patient's posture while the body is in motion
    B. Have the patient perform finger-to-nose, finger-to-finger test, and evaluate the quality of movement
    C. Test the patient's ability to judge distance and speed of movement by drawing a circle
    D. Evaluate the quality of movement control and speed with the patient pointing

159. *You are treating a 16-year-old male diagnosed with chondroma-lacia, degeneration of the patellar surface. The patient is very active and participates in football, basketball, and baseball. Of the following, which exercise would you implement in this patient's treatment program?*
   A. Quadriceps exercise in extension
   B. Short arc quads
   C. Isokinetic, limiting extension to -30°
   D. Exercise bike

160. *A patient is referred to physical therapy for sensory testing. The physician has requested that you evaluate the protective sensa-tions of the patient and implement a treatment program to enhance them. Which of the following would be the most appro-priate test to perform on this patient?*
   A. Deep pressure
   B. Proprioception
   C. Two-point discrimination
   D. Light touch

161. *A new physician on staff refers a patient to physical therapy with a diagnosis of Down's syndrome. Which of the following treat-ments should be implemented in this patient's physical therapy program?*
   A. No specific therapy is necessary for this patient
   B. Range of motion and exercise
   C. Medication
   D. Increase muscle strengthening

162. *You are instructed to perform mobilization on the glenohumeral joint of a patient 6 weeks post heart surgery. You wish to increase abduction of the shoulder for this patient. Which of the following would be the correct mobilization technique?*
   A. Inferior glide
   B. Posterior glide
   C. Anterior glide
   D. Posterior and anterior glide

163. *You are treating a neurological patient in a rehabilitation unit. You are treating the patient according to the theories of Brunnstrom. Which of the following would be an appropriate treatment emphasis according to Brunnstrom?*
    A. Limb synergies are a necessary intermediate stage of recovery and the patient should be encouraged to use limb synergies patterns
    B. Patient should learn diagonal patterns of movement
    C. Do no reinforce abnormal patterns of movement
    D. Do not use associated reactions

164. *You are assessing a patient for a neurological problem as a result of an arterial occlusion in the brain. The patient demonstrates ataxia with severe coordination problems. Which of the following arteries has most likely been occluded in the brain?*
    A. Middle cerebral artery
    B. Posterior cerebral artery
    C. Cerebellar artery
    D. Vertebral artery

165. *You are planning the treatment program for a patient who is referred to physical therapy with Huntington's chorea. This is a hereditary disease that is characterized by irregular movements and tremors. In planning this patient's treatment program, which of the following could a licensed physical therapist perform?*
    A. Advise the physician to prescribe medication to slow down the disease
    B. Advise the patient that there is no treatment; therefore, you are sorry but you cannot help him
    C. Call the family and suggest family education regarding the disease; also contact the social worker for involvement
    D. Utilize postural exercises and balance activities

166. *You are fabricating an orthotic for a patient with a left foot disorder. The patient has a diagnosis of pes planus. The patient will require a longitudinal arch for support and to correct the pes planus. Which of the following shoe modifications would most likely be prescribed for this patient?*

A. Thomas heel
B. Rocker bottom
C. Scaphoid pads
D. Metatarsal bars

167. *A patient is referred to physical therapy with heterotopic bone growth in the quadriceps muscle. The physician has x-rayed the patient and determined that the disease is active. The diagnosis on the script is myositis ossificans. The order is "evaluate and treat." Which of the following treatment programs would be most appropriate for this patient?*
    A. Heat and general exercise
    B. Rest
    C. Exercise bicycle
    D. Treadmill

168. *You are implementing a treatment program for a patient who is 1-day post cesarean delivery. Which of the following would not be an appropriate exercise program on day 1?*
    A. Diaphragmatic breathing
    B. Huffing
    C. Pelvic floor exercises
    D. Leg slides

169. *You have a patient sent from the psychiatric ward to physical therapy for exercise to alleviate his anxiety. When in the clinic the patient becomes withdrawn. The patient occasionally shifts from withdrawal into obscene language, demonstrates very bizarre behavior, and seems to have problems cooperating with physical therapy. Based on these symptoms, which of the following most likely describes the condition of this patient?*
    A. Paranoia
    B. Depression
    C. Schizophrenia
    D. Psychopathy

170. *A patient is referred to physical therapy with an open wound on the lateral malleolus of the right ankle. He is a spinal cord patient who has developed this wound through improper pressure on the ankle. The physician's order is for a lamp to assist in killing the bacteria in the wound and wound healing. In implementing this patient's treatment program, which of the following lamps would be utilized?*
    A. Hot mercury lamp
    B. High-pressure mercury vapor lamp
    C. Low-pressure mercury vapor lamp
    D. Ultraviolet lamp

171. *While performing a musculoskeletal reassessment on a patient you particularly note the end-feel of the glenohumeral joint. The end-feel can be characterized as a hard leather-like stoppage at the end of range of motion. There is full normal range of motion of the shoulder with a slight give at the end. Which of the following best describes the end-feel of this particular patient?*
    A. Bone-to-bone end-feel
    B. Capsular end-feel
    C. Empty end-feel
    D. Springy block end-feel

172. *A patient is sent to physical therapy with an ulnar nerve injury on the right hand. The patient works at a factory sorting various parts for 8 hours a day. The patient is very motivated with rehabilitation and anxious to be aggressive in physical therapy. Which of the following muscles are you going to emphasize with this patient in physical therapy?*
    A. Flexor pollicis longus
    B. Flexor carpi ulnaris
    C. Flexor digitorum superficialis
    D. Flexor carpi radialis

173. *A 60-year-old patient has an injury to the brachial plexus as a result of an automobile accident. Muscle testing shows the patient has a fair minus grade of rhomboids, levator scapulae, and serratus anterior. The physician has determined that the patient has injured the dorsal scapular and long thoracic nerves. Which of the following best describes the origin of injury to the brachial plexus?*
    A. From the rami of the plexus
    B. From the trunks of the plexus
    C. From the lateral cord of the plexus
    D. From the medial cord of the plexus

174. *A patient is a 22-year-old tennis player with a shoulder injury. You are palpating the external rotators of the shoulder. You are palpating the muscle to determine if tenderness or edema exists. The ideal position for palpation of this muscle as it relates to the joint could best be described by which of the following?*
    A. Loose-packed position
    B. Closed-packed position
    C. 20° of movement
    D. 90° of movement

175. *You are evaluating a patient status post cerebrovascular injury. Upon evaluation you note that the patient has the following characteristics: paralysis and weakness on the right side, possible motor apraxia, and a decreased discrimination between left and right. These symptoms describe which of the following?*
    A. Right hemisphere injury
    B. Left hemisphere injury
    C. Cerebellar injury
    D. Brainstem injury

176. *The physician has ordered electrical stimulation to stimulate a denervated muscle. Which of the following types of electrical current would you most likely select to meet this treatment objective?*
    A. Alternating current
    B. High-volt current
    C. Direct current
    D. Interferential stimulation

177. *You are performing goniometric measurement of the shoulder for external rotation. How should the stationary arm of the goniometer be positioned to appropriately measure this patient?*
    A. Longitudinally with the shaft of the ulna
    B. Longitudinally with the styloid process
    C. Parallel or perpendicular to the midline of the floor
    D. Longitudinally over the shaft of the humerus

178. *You are assisting in planning the diet of a runner for a prolonged low-intensity running event. You are determining the number of calories required in the conversion process for energy. The number of calories required is different for protein, carbohydrates, and fats. One gram of carbohydrate yields 4 calories. How many grams of fat would yield 9 calories for this runner?*
    A. 1
    B. 2.25
    C. 3
    D. 4

179. *You are implementing a treatment program of pelvic traction for a patient with a back disorder. Which of the following percentages would cause distraction of the vertebral bodies with lumbar traction?*
    A. 30% of the patient's body weight
    B. 50% of the patient's body weight
    C. 25% of the patient's body weight
    D. 35% of the patient's body weight

180. *A physician has prescribed iontophoresis for a patient with acute inflammation. The chemical ion to be utilized in this case by direct current should be negative. Which of the following chemical ions listed below would be appropriate to use for a negative current?*
    A. Hydrocortisone
    B. Lidocaine
    C. Magnesium
    D. Salicylate

181. *You are determining a treatment program for a weightlifter that injured his quadriceps muscle during a maximal lift. You are interested in performing an eccentric contraction for strengthening. Which of the following exercises would be most appropriate for this patient?*
    A. Lowering a weight during a hard press, performing a negative repetition
    B. Isokinetics
    C. Exercise bicycle
    D. Accelerating the lifting on initiation of movement

182. *A physical therapist is practicing in a rural setting and supervising a physical therapist assistant and a physical therapy aide. The physical therapist will be off for 1 day to attend a continuing education course on preventing low back pain in OB/GYN patients. While the physical therapist is away, the physical therapist assistant will be able to perform all the following duties except?*
    A. Carrying out modified treatment programs
    B. Supervising the physical therapy aide
    C. Evaluating inpatients
    D. Writing progress notes

183. *You are performing a respiratory assessment on a patient for a chest physical therapy program. When reading the chart you are looking at the values of testing performed by the respiratory therapist. One of the particular values that you note is the amount of air that can be forcibly expired by the patient after maximum inspiration. Which of the following was the respiratory therapist evaluating?*
    A. Forced expiratory volume
    B. Forced inspiratory volume
    C. Inspiratory capacity
    D. Tidal volume

184. *Which of the following effects would occur through aerobic exercise in a cardiopulmonary training program for a patient?*
    A. Resting heart rate increases
    B. Cardiac output decreases
    C. Tidal volume decreases
    D. Resting heart rate decreases

185. *You have determined that treating a neurological patient with an exteroceptive stimulation technique would be quite effective in the inhibition of muscles that are extremely spastic. Which of the following techniques listed below would be best in inhibiting the muscles?*

    A. Prolonged icing
    B. Quick icing
    C. Hot packs
    D. Quick stretch

186. *You are performing mobilization on a patient to decrease pain and increase range of motion. It is the patient's first time in the rehabilitation department and you thoroughly explain what to anticipate from the mobilization. You begin by mobilizing the involved side first and comparing it to the uninvolved. Which of the following would not be an absolute contraindication to performing mobilization on this patient?*

    A. Active inflammation
    B. Active infection
    C. Hypermobility
    D. Recent fracture

187. *In implementing a prenatal care program for a patient, which one of the following elements may not be included in her physical therapy regimen?*

    A. Relaxation training
    B. Kegel exercises
    C. Activities of daily living modifications
    D. Valsalva's maneuver

188. *You are treating a patient who has suffered a second-degree collateral ligament injury. The patient injured the knee as a result of a lateral hit during football practice. The patient is currently 2 days post injury. Which of the following is the recommended treatment for a second-degree medial collateral ligament injury?*

    A. Crutch ambulation with toe touch weightbearing
    B. Swimming x 20 minutes, flutter kick only
    C. Exercise bike x 15 minutes
    D. Whirlpool for range of motion

189. *You are implementing a treatment program for a 26-year-old female who is approximately 2 months away from delivering a baby. The patient has been sent to the clinic for low back pain. In implementing a treatment program, which of the following exercises would not be appropriate for this patient to perform.*
   A. Diaphragmatic breathing
   B. Pelvic floor exercise
   C. Partial curl-ups
   D. Postural instructions

190. *This case study involves a spinal cord patient. The patient has the following functional outcomes: vital capacity is 80%, patient is independent with floor to wheelchair transfers, and patient can perform gait with bilateral KAFO and a walker. Based on this information, which of the following is probably the level of lesion of this patient?*
   A. T1 to T5
   B. T9 to T12
   C. L4 to L5
   D. T6 to T8

191. *You are a physical therapist student who is studying the classes of levers in kinesiology. The instructor describes one class of lever in the following way: a common example is a seesaw, or in the body the example would be the atlanto-occipital joint. With the information given above, which of the following is most likely the class of lever described?*
   A. First-class lever
   B. Second-class lever
   C. Third-class lever
   D. Fourth-class lever

192. *You are preparing to perform vibration on a neonate. Which of the following would be a contraindication to performing vibration?*
   A. Persisted fetal circulation
   B. Intolerance to treatment as indicated by low $TcPCO_2$ values
   C. Increased irritability during treatment
   D. Bradycardia

193. You are treating a patient for a lower limb deformity. Upon analyzing the patient's lower extremity, you notice that the distal aspect of the tibia is rotated or twisted medially as compared with its proximal end. Which of the following would best describe this condition?

A. Anteversion
B. Retroversion
C. Internal tibial torsion
D. Genu valgum

194. A physician has ordered whirlpool and debridement to assist in the healing process of a patient with a 2-day-old wound injury. The patient has inflammation as a result of the injury. The layered skin that has been damaged is composed largely of fibrous connective tissue. The nerve fiber and blood vessels are located in this area. Which layer of the tissue has been damaged based on the above description?

A. The epidermis
B. The dermis
C. The subcutaneous layer
D. Adipose cells

195. A patient is sent to physical therapy with a prescription for gait training. The physician has advised you to use a three-point gait pattern with axillary crutch nonweightbearing on the left lower extremity. The patient will need to be measured for correct crutch fitting. Which of the following would be the degree of elbow flexion that would be most desirable for axillary crutches?

A. 10° to 20°
B. 20° to 30°
C. 30°
D. 35°

196. You are performing physical therapy on a retired judge with arthritis in the right hip. After several sessions of heat, ultrasound, and therapeutic exercise, the judge reports that he is feeling the best that he has ever felt. At the end of the session the judge decides to shake your hand and slips you a 20 dollar bill. Which of the following would be proper to do in this situation?

A. Keep the $20 tip and slip it in your pocket
B. Keep the money and place it in the coffee can in the department
C. Explain to the judge that you appreciate his tip but that in a professional relationship, it is unethical for you to accept tips
D. Keep the tip and donate it to a charity

197. *You are performing an evaluation on a patient secondary to a wrist injury from an industrial accident. Upon testing, the patient has a positive Tinel's sign. A positive Tinel's sign would indicate pain over which of the following?*
   A. Severed blood vessel
   B. Severed ligament
   C. Severed muscle
   D. Severed nerve

198. *In a research study, the test yields a statement saying the probability of the distribution obtained occurred by chance alone. This is a statistical test for an association between observed data and expected data represented by frequencies. Which of the following does this define?*
   A. Chi square
   B. Data
   C. T-test
   D. Null hypothesis (HO)

199. *The local community center calls you and asks if you will come over and perform a class on self range of motion to senior citizens to help them maintain their motion. When you go to the geriatric center, which of the following movements would you least likely emphasize?*
   A. Chin tucks
   B. Pectoralis stretch
   C. Hip flexion
   D. Shoulder flexion

200. *You are performing a pediatric assessment for growth and development in a 9-month-old patient. Which of the following should this patient be able to perform?*

    A. The patient should be able to stand and walk holding onto furniture

    B. The patient should be able to sit alone and crawl

    C. The patient should be able to stand and walk unaided

    D. The patient should be able to sit on a small chair

Chapter Nineteen

Sample Test Answers

1.   C. Semimembranosus is the muscle that you would not be evaluating, as it does not insert into the pes anserinus. However, the semimembranosus extends the thigh, and flexes and medially rotates the leg.

   The three muscles that insert into the pes anserinus are the gracilis, sartorius, and semitendinosus. The pes anserinus is located at the medial border of tibial tuberosity. The gracilis adducts the thigh, and flexes and rotates the leg medially. The semitendinosus extends the thigh, flexes and medially rotates the leg.

2.   C. The spring ligament of the foot supports the head of the talipes, which helps to maintain the medial arch of the foot.

   All other statements regarding the spring ligament are false. The long plantar ligament supports the lateral longitudinal arch.

3.   D. The correct answer is hip extension as the inferior gluteal nerve supplies the gluteus maximus muscle. The gluteus maximus muscle is the main extensor of the thigh. Therefore, hip extension would be the motion most likely to be affected to the greatest extent. The superior gluteal nerve supplies the gluteus medius, gluteus minimus, and tensor fasciae latae.

4.   D. The lateral collateral ligament assists in controlling knee rotation and adduction.

   The anterior cruciate ligament prevents anterior displacement of the tibia of the femur. The posterior cruciate ligament prevents posterior displacement of the tibia on the femur. The medial collateral ligament assists in controlling knee rotation and abduction.

5.   D. It is not true that the epiphyseal or growth plate is found in all bones. The epiphyseal or growth plate may only be found in long bones after growth has been completed. It is then replaced by a dense calcified formation known as an epiphyseal line.

6.   B. The bursae are not found in intramuscular locations. Bursae are most likely found where friction is possible, for example between tendons, ligaments, and bones.

7.   C. These three pathologies together are best described as collagen vascular diseases.

   Lupus erythematous is a chronic inflammation disease of the connective tissue, affecting skin, joints, kidney, and nervous system. A butterfly rash is characteristic. Scleroderma is a chronic disease causing sclerosis of the skin and certain organs (eg, lungs, heart, and kidney). Skin is taut, edematous, firmly bound to subcutaneous tissue, and leathery. Dermatomycosis is a skin infection caused by certain fungi.

8.   B. Thromboangiitis obliterans is a disease that involves arteries and veins of the lower extremity. It is characterized by excruciating pain in the leg or foot that is worse at night, decreased sensation, and clamminess and coldness of lower extremity.

   Raynaud's disease involves the fingers. It is characterized by abnormal vasoconstriction of extremities upon exposure to cold or stress. Attacks are characterized by severe blanching of the extremities, followed by cyanosis, then redness, usually with numbness, tingling, and burning. Thrombophlebitis involves a vein disorder, usually in conjunction with formation of a thrombus secondary to inflammation. Pitting edema is a symptom, not a disease.

9.   A. The glenohumeral joint's capsular pattern in a frozen adhesive capsulated shoulder starts with restriction of external rotation, then abduction, followed by internal rotation.

10.   C. The superficial peroneal nerve innervates both the peroneus longus and peroneus brevis.

The deep peroneal nerve innervates the tibialis anterior, peroneus tertius, extensor hallucis longus, extensor digitorum longus, and extensor digitorum brevis.

11. D. Due to its structure and innervation, the cardiac muscle has both atrial and ventricular proportions.

12. C. Cardiac output refers to the amount of blood pumped by the heart in 60 seconds, or 1 minute.

13. B. Mitral stenosis is a lesion in which both stroke volume and pulse pressure would be small.
     Congestive heart failure is an abnormal condition characterized by circulatory congestion caused by cardiac disorders, especially myocardial infarction of the ventricles. Myocardial infarct is an occlusion of a coronary artery that causes myocardial ischemia.

14. B. Myocardial infarctions most frequently occur in the left ventricle as a result of occlusion to the left coronary artery.

15. D. Thrombosis, or thrombi, is the most common cause of stroke in older adults because of sclerotic tissue/vessels.
     Aneurysm is a localized dilatation of the wall of a blood vessel, generally caused by atherosclerosis and hypertension. Hemorrhaging is bleeding externally or internally. Thrombosis is an abnormal vascular condition in which thrombus develops within a blood vessel of the body.

16. A. The action of digitalis on a patient with congestive heart failure is to decrease the heart rate and increase strength of the contraction.

17. D. A concussion may best be defined as a temporary state of paralysis of the nervous function. This will usually result in loss of consciousness following a blow to the head or head trauma.

18. C. In a patient who has had rheumatoid arthritis for a long peri-
     od of time, a common symptom would be ulnar deviation of the
     fingers.
        Rheumatoid arthritis is a systemic disease, characterized by
     painful joints, tenderness, inflammation, swelling, redness, heat,
     fibrous adhesions, morning stiffness, and proliferation of granu-
     lation tissue known as pannus.
        Osteoarthritis is characterized by stiffness, pain, roughened
     surface, narrowing of joint spaces, and weightbearing joints.

19. C. The etiology of arthritis is degeneration caused by aging. It is
     a degenerative joint disease of articular cartilage.
        Gout is a form of arthritis in which sodium urate crystals are
     deposited near or in the joint. It is common in the great toe.

20. B. The anatomical dead space is best defined as the area occupied
     by the airways which does not permit gas exchange.

21. D. It is an untrue statement that the strength/duration curve
     exhibits development and fatigue during a prolonged stimulus.
     Strength/duration curve is utilized in testing for nerve degenera-
     tion and regeneration. It will also show the relationship of the
     stimulus intensity to duration in reaching an excitation threshold.

22. C. In regard to energy for muscle contractions, it is false that
     energy may be stored as creatine phosphate. All other statements
     are true.

23. D. The most distinctive feature of diabetes mellitus versus dia-
     betes insipidus is that diabetes insipidus is associated with a pitu-
     itary disease, typically a tumor in the pituitary, while diabetes
     mellitus is associated with the pancreas.

24. C. The period between the 21st and the 40th day of gestation is
     the time during prenatal development when the cardiovascular
     system is beginning its development and is most at risk.

25. B. When skin is damaged by excessive exposure to heat, the first stage is inflammation. Inflammation is a response to the injury or stress in which blood vessels dilate and become more permeable.

26. B. Disadvantages of isotonic exercise: loads muscle at the weakest point, momentum factor in lifting, does not develop accuracy at functional speeds.

27. C. The frontal lobe carries out the functions of personality and speech, as well as intelligence and motor activities.

Vision is the responsibility of the occipital lobe. Sensory perception and interpretation are the responsibility of the parietal lobe. Hearing and speech are the responsibility of the temporal lobe.

28. A. Vision and interpretation of visual data.

29. B. The axillary nerve would most likely be injured since it is in the location of the shoulder. Some fibers of the nerve also supply the capsule of the shoulder joint.

The others would not be involved since they are located distally to the shoulder.

30. C. Spina bifida myelocele is the most severe form of spina bifida.

Soft tissue contained in the meninges describes spina bifida meningocele. Soft tissue contained in the spinal cord describes spina bifida myelomeningocele. A herniated sac contained in the spinal cord describes spina bifida syringomyelocele. Spina bifida occulta is a defective closure of the laminae of the vertebral column in the lumbosacral region without hernial protrusion of the spinal cord or meninges.

31. A. With a lesion of the lateral cord brachial plexus, you would expect to find paralysis of the biceps, coracobrachialis, and the finger flexors.

Paralysis of the deltoid would most likely be a result of an axillary nerve lesion. Paralysis of the wrist extension would be a result of the axillary nerve and the radial nerve. Paralysis of the hand intrinsic would involve the medial cord of the brachial plexus.

32. B. Most helpful for this patient would be to teach him or her rhythmic initiation. The patient would know how to initiate movement in using trunk control for transfers. This technique would help the patient to initiate movement from supine to sit or from left to right sidelying through using the trunk to roll.

33. A. Alveoli are the sites of gas exchange in the pulmonary system. Alveoli consist of small outpouching of walls of alveolar space through which gas exchange takes place between alveolar air and pulmonary capillary blood.

34. C. Passive range of motion will affect pulmonary ventilation depending upon the number of joints involved.

35. A. Asthma will result in episodes of dyspnea, difficulty in breathing, "air hunger," and difficulty in expiration.

36. C. Common pressure points in the sidelying position include the ears, shoulders, ribs, greater trochanter, medial and lateral condyles, and the ankles.

37. A. Loose-packed position is when the joint is in a resting position where the joint's range of motion is under the least amount of stress. The maximum loose-packed position for the ankle joint would be 10° plantar flexion, midway between inversion and eversion.

38. D. A disadvantage of a cemented hip is that it does require more bone tissue removal.
     Advantages of a cemented hip would be that it allows for early weightbearing, surgeons report a 90% success rate, and there is less postoperative pain.

39. C. When the elbow joint is in midposition or semiprone, the joint will have the greatest advantage for optimum force output.

40. D. The combined action of the tendinous cuff muscles (SITS) would produce depression of the head of the humerus in the joint.

41. C. For a paraplegic, prolonged standing with braces in a lordotic position would result in stretching of the hip extensors and iliofemoral ligament.

42. C. The axis motion that the radial and ulnar deviation lies in would be the sagittal plane through the capitate. All other answers are incorrect.

43. B. Tensor fasciae latae would be the muscle responsible for tightness that would result in the hip joint remaining abducted and slightly flexed when lowered to the table. The tensor fasciae latae is one of the 10 muscles of the gluteal region, arising from the outer lip of the iliac crest, the iliac spine, and the deep fasciae latae (also called tensor fascia femoris).

     Psoas major acts to flex and laterally rotate the thigh and to flex and laterally bend the spine. Semitendinosus functions to flex the leg and rotate it medially after flexion and to extend the thigh. Rectus femoris functions to flex the leg.

44. A. Normal expansion at the xiphoid process should measure approximately 5 to 10 cm.

45. C. A patient with pronated feet would demonstrate eversion of the calcaneus with a medial weight line. All other answers are incorrect.

46. C. Heberden's node is an abnormal cartilaginous or bony enlargement most frequently located in the distal interphalangeal joint of a finger, usually occurring in degenerative diseases of the joints.

47. D. The hamstring muscle is any one of three muscles at the back of the thigh: medially, the semimembranosus and the semitendinosus; and laterally, the biceps femoris. The hamstring is most active during midswing to deceleration.

48. C. Iliac crest is the most likely landmark to use in palpation of the L4 region.

49. B. You would expect weakness in the motor activities of wrist flexion, finger extension, and elbow extension. You would not expect weakness in finger flexion because with a C7 nerve root impingement you would expect finger flexion motor activities to be intact and not involved.

50. D. In performing ultrasound under water, the most important safety feature is to have a ground fault interruption circuit so that the patient cannot be accidentally electrocuted.

51. D. The first priority in dealing with a newly admitted burn patient is to begin wound cleaning, debridement, and sterile dressing. Sterile whirlpool is used in order to promote healing, control infection, and aid in loosening necrotic tissue, and making debridement easier. Sterile towels and dressing must also be used post whirlpool. It is extremely important to maintain a faultless sterile technique so that no cross infections occur.

52. C. When administering ultrasound under water, the sound head should be placed approximately 1 inch from the area to be treated, which in this case is the medial arch of the foot.

53. A. Hip flexion would not be an emphasis in a geriatric program, as typically this is not a limited range of motion seen in that age group. All other areas would be emphasized to reduce the limitations experienced by these patients.

54. C. Tibialis anterior, peroneus tertius, and extensor hallucis longus are muscles that are active during the swing phase, acceleration stage. These muscles remain active throughout the entire stage to help shorten the extremity so it can clear the ground by holding the ankle in a neutral position.

55. C. During the swing phase, deceleration stage, the hamstring muscles contract to slow down the swing phase just prior to heel strike, thus permitting the heel to strike quietly in a controlled manner.

56. B. With an impacted fracture there is a bone break in which the adjacent fragmented ends of the bone are wedged together.

   With a displaced fracture, a traumatic bone break takes place in which two ends of a fractured bone are separated from each other. An intraarticular fracture involves the articular surfaces of a joint.

57. B. The normal conduction pathway for muscular contraction of the heart to follow is the right atrium, to the left atrium, to the ventricles.

58. A. The sinus node, an area of specialized heart tissue, is located in the right atrium of the heart.

59. C. Pectus carinatum is best described as a sternum that is displaced anteriorly with increasing anterior posterior diameter.

60. D. The brachioradialis is responsible for forearm pronation, supination, and elbow flexion. Therefore, if the patient has an injury in the brachioradialis muscles, those movements would now be limited.

61. B. Flexor carpi ulnaris, which functions to flex and adduct the hand, does not have dual innervation.

   Flexor digitorum profundus, flexor pollicis brevis, and the lumbricales all have dual innervation by the median nerve and the ulnar nerve.

62. D. With a patient who has an injury involving the tibialis muscles, you can expect to have a deep peroneal nerve involved, as that is what innervates the anterior tibialis muscle.

63. C. The group of muscles that attaches to the ischial tuberosity are as follows: semimembranosus, biceps femoris, and semitendinosus.

64. C. The biceps correspond with the C5 reflex.

   The brachioradialis corresponds with C6. The triceps corresponds with C7.

65.   C. The facial nerve is the correct answer because the patient has a diagnosis of Bell's palsy. Bell's palsy is a condition that causes paralysis of the facial nerve.

66.   D. Flexor carpi ulnaris does not assist in pronation of the radioulnar joint. Muscles active in pronation include brachioradialis, pronator teres, pronator quadratus, and flexor carpi radialis.

67.   B. The median nerve innervates the second and third digits of the hand.
      The ulnar nerve is responsible for the fourth and fifth digits.

68.   A. A characteristic that is not typically seen with an upper motor neuron lesion is muscle atrophy. A patient with an upper motor neuron lesion typically has spasticity, hyperreflexia, and Babinski sign is possible.

69.   B. Lactic acid build-up following exercise will cause muscle fatigue.
      Glycogen and glucose are fuels used for exercise.

70.   D. Maximum heart rate is calculated by 220 minus age. This number can be used to help determine target heart rate at which you want the patient to exercise when it is multiplied by 60% to 90%, depending on the level of exercise desired.

71.   C. It would be indicative of hypertension if blood pressure readings were above 140/90. Typically, hypertension is indicated when three different readings are all 140/90 or above.

72.   A. The radial nerve, which is the largest branch of the brachial plexus, arising on each side as a continuation of the posterior cord, is the nerve that passes through the anatomical snuffbox of the wrist. Therefore, if you were evaluating a patient who might have suffered an injury to the nerve crossing the anatomical snuffbox, you would evaluate the radial nerve.

The median nerve is one of the terminal branches of the brachial plexus that extends along the radial portions of the fore-arm and hand and supplies various muscles and the skin of these parts. The ulnar nerve is one of the terminal branches of the brachial plexus that arises on each side from the medial cord of the plexus. The musculocutaneous nerve is one of the terminal branches of the brachial plexus.

73. B. At the subtalar joint of the ankle, eversion and inversion movements take place.

74. B. The radial nerve would most likely be injured, as it is in the closest proximity to the distal radius.

75. C. The carpometacarpal joint in the thumb is unique in that it is classified as a saddle joint. A saddle joint permits no axial rota-tion but allows flexion, extension, adduction, and abduction.

   The uniaxial joint is a synovial joint in which movement is only in one axis as with a pivot or hinge joint. A hinge joint is a synovial joint providing a connection in which articular surfaces are closely molded together in a manner that permits extension motion in one place.

76. D. Origin is the proximal attachment of a limb muscle.

   Tendon, one of many white, glistening fibrous bands of tissue that attach muscle to bone, refers to the tendinous structure. Insertion is the distal attachment of the muscle. The belly is the belly part of the muscle.

77. A. Electromyogram helps in diagnosing neuromuscular problems by applying surface electrodes or by inserting a needle electrode into the muscle and observing electric activity with an oscillo-scope and a loudspeaker.

   Arthroscopy is the examination of the interior of a joint, per-formed by inserting a specially designed endoscope through a small incision. An EKG (electrocardiogram) is a graphic record produced by an electrocardiograph. A myelogram is an x-ray film taken after injection of a radiopaque medium into the subarach-noid space to demonstrate any distortions of the spinal cord, spinal nerve roots, and subarachnoid space.

78. B. The midbrain, one of the three parts of the brainstem and lying below the cerebrum and just above the pons, is not considered one of the three major brain regions.

   The three major divisions of the brain region are (1) brainstem, which is the portion of the brain comprising the medulla oblongata, the pons, and the mesencephalon; (2) cerebellum, the part of the brain located in the posterior cranial fossa behind the brainstem; (3) cerebrum, the largest and uppermost section of the brain divided by a central sulcus into the left and right cerebral hemispheres.

79. A. The Valsalva maneuver is a forced expiratory effort against a closed airway, as when an individual holds his or her breath and tightens the muscles in a strenuous effort to move a heavy object or to change position in bed. In pregnancy, the Valsalva maneuver both increases pressure on the pelvic diaphragm and causes fluctuations in venous return to the heart.

80. A. The main function of erythrocytes, also known as red blood cells, is to transport oxygen in the body. Erythrocytes are biconcave discs that contain hemoglobin confined within a lipid membrane. Erythrocytes originate in the marrow of the long bones.

81. A. The stimulus for testing flexor withdrawal is applied to the sole of the foot with the lower extremity in extended position to start.

82. A. An increase in extensor tone occurs when the patient's position is supine for the tonic labyrinthine reflex. No specific stimulus is required and the response is dependent upon patient positioning. Prone increases flexor tone, sidelying increases extensor tone, and the other sidelying limb increases flexor tone in the nonweightbearing limb.

83. C. A positive response to bouncing a patient several times on the soles of the feet but not allowing his or her to bear weight is increased flexor tone in the lower extremities.

84. C. An incorrect or untrue statement regarding a cerebral palsy child would be that the child can hold or bring the head into a normal position. Typically, a cerebral palsy child cannot hold or bring the head into a normal position. Such children cannot support themselves. Typically, they will demonstrate a scissors gait pattern. They will usually have an exaggerated reflex response. They may be classified as either spastic, ataxic, or athetoid. They may be either passive or stiff and cannot adjust the body position.

85. C. A malingerer is one who pretends to be ill to arouse sympathy or who intentionally slows recuperation from a disorder to continue to receive insurance benefits or other emotional, or social benefits from the disorder. If the physical therapist suspects the patient is a malingerer, he or she should discuss the case in a teamwork approach and notify the physician.

    Negligence is failure to do what another reasonable practitioner would have done under similar circumstances. A hypochondriac is a person with a chronic, abnormal concern about his or her health. A paranoid patient has a mental disorder characterized by an impaired sense of reality and persistent delusions.

86. D. Four-point gait pattern is a slow, stable gait pattern of left crutch, right leg, right crutch, left leg.

    A three-point gait involves nonweightbearing sequence. The crutch advances first, then the uninvolved leg, then the crutch. A two-point gait requires more balance. The opposite crutch and leg advance simultaneously. A swing-through is used when both lower extremities are involved and a patient swings the crutches, then hops on one leg.

87. A. Allograft is the transfer of skin between the same species. It could involve a cadaver skin.

    An autograft is grafted skin from the same individual. A heterograft is a graft from an animal (eg, a pig). Z-plasty is a surgical revision of a scar or closure of a wound using a Z-shaped incision to reduce contractures of the adjacent skin.

88. D. Slump test is utilized to determine whether an impingement of the nerve root is sustained in the thoracic lumbar region.

Compression test is utilized to test for neurological pathology in the cervical spine at any level. Distraction test determines the effectiveness of traction, which may be used to alleviate pain. This is a complementary test to the compression test, as it is used to obtain the reverse effect. Ely's test checks the L2 to L4 nerve root lever for impingement or for tightness of the rectus femoris.

89. D. A vertebrobasilar artery involvement will result in loss of consciousness, as well as the patient being comatose or in a vegetative state. The patient will have no ability to speak and may have either hemiplegia or quadriplegia.

90. D. Medication is not required to be listed in an initial evaluation according to the APTA *Standards of Care*.

91. B. Maintaining joint mobility through exercise and stretching, heat, and postural instructions is the best treatment for a patient with Marie-Strumpell disease (also named ankylosing spondylitis).

92. D. Deep pressure test is the least important when testing a patient for peripheral vascular disease.

When testing a patient for peripheral vascular disease, the following would all be appropriate: rubor test, girth measurements, volumetric measurement, reactive hyperemia, and ischemia test.

93. D. Subscapularis is not a muscle that attaches to the greater tuberosity of the humerus but to the lesser tuberosity of the humerus.

Supraspinatus, infraspinatus, and teres minor attach to the greater tuberosity of the humerus.

94. B. The most appropriate treatment to begin post surgery is massage. This would be correctly performed by doing the proximal segment first.

You would not change the physician's orders by substituting Jobst compression pump for massage without consultation with the physician. You would proceed with ordering a garment for the patient if necessary.

95.   D. When a patient questions you regarding a procedure performed by the physician, it would be appropriate to have the patient consult with the physician. Instruct him or her that you are not able to provide that information.

96.   A. The typical treatment temperature for paraffin is 50°C.
       The conversion to Fahrenheit is as follows:
       Fahrenheit = (temperature in Celsius x 9/5 + 32).
       Therefore, temperature in Fahrenheit is 50 x 9 = 450, divided by 5, which is 90 + 32 or 122°F.

97.   A. The major components of a problem-oriented medical record are subjective, objective, assessment, and plan.

98.   A. Subjective data collection is the process in which data relating to the patient's problem is elicited from the patient. A patient who states that his chief concern is limited movement or loss of range of motion in the left shoulder is stating his own perception versus something that may be evaluated by objective standards. Therefore, this information should be placed under subjective in the SOAP note format.

99.   C. A disorder characterized by the growth of cartilage in the epiphyses of the long bones resulting in the limbs remaining short and is transmitted as an autosomal dominant gene, is achondroplasia.
       Osteogenesis imperfecta is a genetic disorder involving defective development of the connective tissue. It is inherited as an autosomal dominant trait and is characterized by abnormally brittle and fragile bones that are easily fractured by the slightest trauma. Typically, the patient presents with multiple fractures with minimal trauma. Fibrous dysplasia pertains to displacement of the osseous tissue within the affected bones. Bone tumor is any abnormal growth of new tissue, benign or malignant.

100. D. Fibrous dysplasia is not another name for thyrotoxicosis, as this pertains to an abnormal condition characterized by the fibrous displacement of the osseous tissue within the affected bones.

    Grave's disease, as well as primary and secondary hyperthyroidism, is also called thyrotoxicosis. The condition of hyperthyroidism is typically caused by secretions of the thyroid gland, which increases the basal metabolism rate, causing an increased demand for food to support metabolic activities.

101. D. Interferential current stimulation is best described as a medium-frequency current, approximately 4000 Hz, which typically utilizes four electrodes in a crossed pattern on the patient. It is primarily used for pain relief and muscle spasms.

    Russian stimulation involves stimulation in the midrange frequency, typically 2400 to 2500 Hz. High-volt electric stimulation is typically set up with a rate of 50 to 120 Hz per 10- to 30-minute period for acute pain.

102. A. Transcutaneous electrical nerve stimulation is the only type of stimulation that the patient can utilize 24 hours a day. The patient is set up in independent use of a TENS unit to assist in alleviating pain.

103. B. Gluteus medius, gluteus minimum, and tensor fasciae latae are all muscles of hip abduction and their nerve innervation is the superior gluteal nerve. Inferior gluteal nerve is innervation for gluteus maximus.

    Psoas major, iliacus, and sartorius have innervation from the femoral nerve and the lumbar plexus. Gluteus medius, gluteus minimus, and sartorius have innervation from the superior gluteal nerve and femoral nerve. Gluteus medius, gracilis, and pectineus have innervation from the femoral nerve and the superior gluteal nerve.

104. D. The femoral, obturator, and inferior gluteal nerves are the correct answer, as the hip adductor muscles consist of the pectineus, gracilis, adductor longus, adductor brevis, and adductor magnus. Their innervation includes the inferior gluteal nerve for the gluteus maximus, the femoral nerve for the pectineus, and the obturator nerve for the adductor brevis, adductor longus, adductor magnus, and gracilis.

105. D. Evaporative coolants or a spray not significantly lower tissue temperature below the surface. Evaporative coolants cause a chemical reaction that produces a cool feeling on the outside surface of the skin.

Ice massage, cryopressure, and ice towels all decrease swelling by decreasing tissue temperature.

106. C. Iontophoresis is a modality in which chemical substances are entered into the body with a direct current to decrease inflammation.

Myoflex with ultrasound, phonophoresis, and ultrasound are treatments that may decrease inflammation but are not chemical substances placed into the body with a direct current.

107. B. Convection is the transfer of heat energy by combining mechanisms of fluid and conduction (eg, diathermy, paraffin).

Conversion does not exist. Conduction is heat transferred from one part of the body to another through molecular collision (eg, hot packs). Radiation is heat transferred in the form of electromagnetic waves without heating the intervening medium (eg, warming by the sun).

108. D. Grave-five mobilization is an example of a manual therapy technique that could not be performed by a physical therapist. Typically, it is performed by a physician with a patient under anesthesia. It is a manipulation of such force that it breaks the entire joint from being frozen. Grade-five mobilization is defined as a thrusting movement done at the anatomical limits of the joint.

109. D. Saunders cervical traction device is recommended for a patient with temporomandibular joint dysfunction (TMJ). The Saunders cervical traction device does not contact the jaw, thereby reducing further aggravation of the temporomandibular joints.

    Conventional cervical traction methods utilize head halters that fit under the chin anteriorly and on the occipital bone posteriorly. Even when care is taken to minimize the force on the chin, there is sufficient force to cause an undesirable effect on the temporomandibular joints.

110. D. Intermittent mechanical traction is described as intermittent traction when there is typically a hold and rest period.

    Autotraction utilizes a special traction bench made up of two sections that can be individually angled and rotated. The patient applies traction by pulling with his or her own arms. With gravity lumbar traction, the lower border and the circumference of the rib cage are anchored through a specially made vest secured to the top of the bed. The patient is placed on a bed that is tilted vertically, putting the patient in a position in which the free weight of the legs and hips exerts a traction force on the lumbar spine by gravity. With manual traction, the therapist grasps the patient and manually applies a traction force either for a few seconds or by a sudden, quick thrust.

111. C. A patient with paranoia would exhibit psychotic behavior, appearing suspicious, resentful, and rigid.

    Hypochondria is a disorder characterized by a chronic, abnormal concern about health. Hysteria is a state of tension or excitement characterized by unmanageable fear and temporary loss of control over the emotions. Depression is an emotional state characterized by feelings of sadness, despair, emptiness, and hopelessness.

112. B. A patient with depression would appear pessimistic, irritable, lack self-confidence, and have a gloomy outlook on life.

    A psychopath is a person who has an antisocial personality disorder. Schizophrenia is any one of a large group of psychotic disorders characterized by a gross distortion of reality, disturbances of communication, withdrawal from social interaction, and disorganized and fragmented thought, perception, and emotional reaction.

113. C. Hypertonia is a condition characterized by excessive tone in the limbs, which are resistant to both active and passive movement.

   Flaccidity is characterized by weak, soft, and flabby muscles, that lack normal muscle tone. Hypotonia is characterized by less than adequate muscle contractions and a state of decreased motor neuron excitability. Rigidity is a condition of hardness, stiffness, or inflexibility.

114. C. At level C6, a patient can provide independent pressure relief. This is the minimal level of injury a patient can have in order to be able to provide independent care.

   At level C4, a patient is able only to direct pressure-relief activities. At level C5, a patient is able to assist in manual wheelchair pressure relief. At level C8, a patient is independent in pressure relief including wheelchair, and push-ups.

115. A. The minimal level a patient can have to perform self range of motion independently is C7.

   At C4 and C5, a patient can only direct range of motion. At C7 and C8, a patient is independent in range of motion.

116. B. Sacral sparing occurs when the patient has paralysis and loss of sensation except in the sacral area.

   Cauda equina injury involves the lower end of the spinal cord at the first lumbar vertebra and the bundle of lumbar, sacral, and coccygeal nerve roots that emerge from the spinal cord and descend through the spinal canal of the sacrum and coccyx. Central cord syndrome occurs when there is damage to the central portion of the cord and an incomplete lesion. Typically, greater deficits are found in the upper extremities than the lower extremities upon evaluation. Brown-Sequard syndrome is a traumatic neurologic disorder resulting from compression of one side of the spinal cord, typically seen after a knife-type injury. There is also an incomplete lesion, which typically results in loss of motor function on the same side as the lesion and loss of pain and temperature on the opposite side.

117. B. Scleroderma is a relatively rare autoimmune disease affecting the blood vessels and connective tissue. It is characterized by fibrous degeneration of the connective tissue of the skin, lungs, and internal organs.

Chronic contractures are an abnormal condition of a joint, characterized by flexion and fixation. Fibrositis is an inflammation of fibrous connective tissue, usually characterized by a poorly defined set of symptoms, including pain and stiffness of the neck, shoulder, and trunk. Myositis is an inflammation of muscle tissue, usually of the voluntary muscles.

118. C. Normal alignment of a patient from the lateral view would be the head in neutral position with the scapula flat against the upper back, and the shoulder in neutral position with the plumb line falling through the shoulder joint.

Normal alignment from the posterior view would be the head in neutral position, scapula in neutral position, level alignment in comparison to each other, with the plumb line falling straight through the thoracic and lumbar spine.

119. B. Functional performance of the lower extremity requires that a patient have a muscle grade of fair plus.

120. A. A muscle grade of poor is defined as production of movement only in a gravity-eliminated position.

A muscle grade of trace would be no movement but palpable twitching of the muscle contraction. A muscle grade of fair would be production of movement against gravity. A muscle grade of zero would be no palpable muscle contraction.

121. D. Testing bilaterally starting with the injured side first is an incorrect method of performing manual muscle testing. When performing manual muscle testing, it is appropriate to test bilaterally starting on the noninjured side and then comparing to the injured side.

All other answers listed would be important in performing manual muscle testing. The following considerations should be followed when performing manual muscle tests: (1) test bilaterally starting with the noninjured side; (2) isolate the muscle you are testing, line up the origin and insertion; (3) palpate the muscle testing for contraction; (4) stabilize the proximal part—you must know proper hand position to isolate the muscle you are testing; (5) apply the correct amount of resistance for testing strength and, to receive maximum cooperation from the patient, inform him or her of the treatment you are performing.

122. A. 36° is the correct temperature conversion from Fahrenheit to Celsius. This is performed by the following:
Celsius = (temperature in Fahrenheit − 32) x 5/9
(98°F − 32) = 66 x 5 = 330/9 = 36°C

123. C. Agonist is a term defined as a muscle group whose contraction is considered to be the principal agent in producing a joint motion.
Antagonist is defined as a muscle group that is noncontracting and passively elongates or shortens to permit the motion to occur. Concentric refers to a shortening in the contraction. Eccentric refers to elongation of the muscle during contraction.

124. C. Inverse square law states that the intensity of radiation from a light source varies inversely to the square of the distance from the source. Clinical application means the further the infrared light, for example, is moving from the patient, the greater the decrease in intensity will be

125. B. A patient in a coma would show no voluntary movement, be unresponsive to stimulus, have no reflexes, and exhibit a positive Babinski response.
The aftereffect of a cerebrovascular accident depends on the location and extent of ischemia. Paralysis, weakness, speech defect, aphasia, and even death may occur. Patients in a stupor would exhibit a state of lethargy and unresponsiveness in which they seem unaware of their surroundings.

126. A. A patient should only be seen once a week when receiving a third-degree erythemal dosage, which can produce tissue damage.

Following is a chart of the appropriate treatment frequency for a patient:

Suberythemal dosage	Daily
Second-degree erythemal dosage	Two times a week
Third-degree erythemal dosage	Once a week
Fourth-degree erythemal dosage	Once every 3 to 4 months

127. A. Standard deviation of the mean plus or minus one is graded based on the score of 68% of the students.

128. D. In order to perform an ethical research study, prior to starting the research a patient should sign the informed consent document.

Informing the patient that he or she has the right to terminate the experiment at any time, debriefing the patient following the experiment, and explaining the end results of the experiment to the patient are necessary for a study to be ethical. However, an informed consent document must be signed first.

129. C. The most appropriate exercise for a patient in early stages of rehabilitation after a nonsurgical operation would be closed-chain isokinetic exercise such as a stair machine.

130. D. The American Red Cross has recently recommended calling 911 (EMS) before instituting CPR, because if the adult has suffered cardiac arrest, he will need defibrillation immediately to increase his chance of survival.

131. B. The social worker should be contacted to start discharge planning in cooperation with the patient, family, and physical therapist.

The physician has already given you the order for discharge so it is not necessary to contact him or her first. The home health agency can be contacted later through the social worker. The patient's family will also be contacted by the social worker in a team approach. Therefore, the social worker would be the correct person to contact first to get the ball rolling.

132. A. Bleeding should receive the first consideration if the patient has a wound. Direct pressure should be applied to stop bleeding.

With shock, body temperature should be kept normal; extreme variations of temperature will accentuate the condition of shock. The correct body position should be arranged with the head and trunk level and the lower limbs elevated. Lastly, oxygen, if available, should be administered.

133. A. Strengthening for bed mobility for a C6 quadriplegic should emphasize the pectoralis major. The pectoralis major serves to flex, adduct, and medially rotate the arm in the shoulder joint.

134. A. Given the information provided in this question, the patient is most likely experiencing heat cramps. Heat cramps are caused by depletion of both water and salt because of heat exhaustion. They usually occur after vigorous physical exertion in an extremely hot environment or under other conditions causing profuse sweating.

Heat syncope results in weakness, fatigue, and loss of motor tone. The patient typically will have blurred vision and an elevated body temperature. Heat exhaustion results in fatigue, weakness, incoordination, and elevated body temperature. With heat hyperpyrexia, the patient becomes irrational, with muscle flaccidity and involuntary limb movements, as well as seizures.

135. A. When the stimulus is flexing the head, the positive reaction will result in arm flexion and leg extension.

If the test stimulus had been extending the patient's head, the positive response would then have been arm extension and leg flexion.

136. C. Utilizing the Rule of Nines, an anterior arm is assigned a value of 4.5% and an anterior leg a value of 9.0%. Therefore, the correct answer would be 13.5%.

137. C. A Knight-Taylor spinal brace is utilized for fractures above the L3 region and is a rigid, high-back brace.

Lumbar corsets are made from canvas or cloth and are not utilized with a fracture. A Taylor spinal brace is a semirigid brace that is used in thoracic and lumbar spine disease. A Jewett brace is a three-point brace that prevents hyperextension.

138. B. Utilizing the Rule of Nines, the percentage of burns listed for a child's arm is 9% and for the leg 14%, so the correct answer is 23%.

139. B. A resting hand splint is a static splint for wrist and hands which is typically utilized with arthritic patients. It is designed to support the hand in a functional position.

    A wrist cock-up splint immobilizes the wrist but allows full range of motion in MCP flexion and thumb opposition and is utilized for inflammation. A static wrist splint immobilizes the wrist for protection. An ulnar/radial gutter is designed to control radial/ulnar deviation of the wrist.

140. B. Shoulder splints are used to immobilize the shoulder to promote healing of a brachial plexus injury. They can be designed to be placed in any degree of motion that is appropriate for optimal healing.

    A shoulder sling is designed to support the elbow but does not rest the shoulder for brachial plexus injury. An elbow splint is used to immobilize and protect the elbow. In the case of brachial plexus injury, you want some immobilization; you do not want free active range of motion constantly.

141. D. Pistoning of the socket is a gait deviation as a result of poor socket fit, weak suspension, and overly soft knee friction.

    Lateral whip is generally caused by a knee bolt alignment that is too medial. Rotation of the foot in heel strike is usually a result of too much toe-out or resistance on the heel cushion or plantar flexion bumper. Instability of the knee is most commonly caused by a plantar flexion resistance that is too high.

142. C. An antalgic gait results when a patient will not bear weight on the injured lower extremity.

    Steppage gait results in the patient lifting the knee very high to clear the foot. Foot slap occurs when the patient has a weak or absent dorsiflexor and the foot slaps down on the ground. Abducted lurch occurs when the patient leans over the hip to place the center of gravity over the hip. It is a compensatory technique for a gluteus medius muscle weakness.

143. A. The first step in performing an educational program to a company with repetitive motion injuries is to instruct the personnel in proper warm-up and stretching exercises as a prevention technique.

144. C. The most appropriate immediate treatment for a burn patient is passive range of motion in extension, as well as emphasizing position of the elbow in full extension. This is done to prevent flexion contractures.

   Depending upon the extent of the burn, whirlpool may be ordered for debridement.

145. D. To perform proper chest physical therapy on the right middle lobe, the patient should be in the left sidelying position, rotated one-half turn backward, with the bed elevated 14 inches. Pillows may be placed under the right hip, and percussion should be performed on the right side at nipple level.

146. A. You should contact the patient's family and request that they come to the hospital. It is important for the patient to have support personnel there while being instructed in transfers into and out of a vehicle. If possible, use the actual vehicle in which the patient will be transported.

147. C. When treating a wound patient, the least important to note in the progress notes is the strength of the hip muscles since you are primarily focusing on the wound and rehabilitation of wound healing.

148. D. A correct example is dressing and undressing. This is one of the activities of daily living that would help retrain the patient in a functional activity.

149. B. Pulmonary edema produces dull percussion sounds with wheezing and crackling upon auscultation.

   Atelectasis will produce dull percussion sounds and decreased breath sounds with auscultation. Pneumonia will produce dull percussion sounds, decreased breath sounds, and sounds of a pleural lung. Pneumothorax will result in hyperresonance, and increased breath sounds.

150. A. When treating a patient 3 days postoperative, it would be appropriate for the patient to have monitored ambulation with no symptoms.

   Lower extremity ergometry x 15 or x 30 minutes, and upper extremity ergometry x 15 minutes would be too aggressive to start on a patient 3 days post cardiac surgery.

151. B. Proprioception tests the patient's ability to determine the direct position sense.

   Kinesthesia tests the patient's ability to determine movement sensation. Graphesthesia tests the ability of a patient to recognize letters and numbers written on the patient's skin. Barognosis is the ability to determine the weight of an object.

152. D. Proper body mechanics for a post cesarean patient would be to get up from a lying down position by rolling over to the side, swinging the legs over the edge, and getting up slowly.

   When sitting, the patient should avoid soft chairs, as they are hard to get up from and have poor back support. When standing, the patient should keep the chin in and contract the abdominal muscles. When bending over, the patient should keep a curve in the low back with one foot in front of the other.

153. B. The upper abdominal reflex test involves thoracic 8, 9, 10.

   The lower abdominal reflex test involves thoracic 10, 11, 12.

154. A. Bell's palsy is a paralysis of the facial nerve resulting from trauma to the nerve, compression of the nerve by a tumor, or possibly, an unknown infection. The typical treatment is electrical stimulation direct current to the motor points of the facial muscles.

155. C. Teaching proper body mechanics is a psychomotor area that deals with motor skills.

   Educational contacts are usually divided into three areas. First is cognitive, which deals with the information area; second is psychomotor, which deals with the motor skills; and third is affective, which deals with feelings.

156. B. An appropriate treatment program for a pediatric patient with cystic fibrosis would include both breathing exercises and postural drainage. This would be the most aggressive form of treatment for this patient that can be performed by a licensed physical therapist.

157. B. A patient with a capsular pattern of the hip will exhibit first a decreased range of motion in flexion, then abduction, then internal rotation.

158. A. Observation of the patient's posture while the body is in motion is an example of a dynamic balance equilibrium coordination test.

   Having the patient perform a finger-to-nose, finger-to-finger test to evaluate the quality of movement, testing the patient's ability to judge distance and speed of movement by drawing a circle, and evaluating the quality of movement control and speed with the patient pointing are examples of nonequilibrium coordination.

159. A. The most effective form of treatment for chondromalacia would involve performing quadriceps exercises in extension so no further degeneration of the patellar surface would occur.

160. D. Light touch would be appropriate to perform on a patient to determine if the protective sensations are in place.

   Deep pressure, proprioception, and two-point discrimination are examples of discriminative sensations.

161. A. Typically, no specific type of physical therapy is ordered for a patient with Down's syndrome. The diagnosis of Down's syndrome does not indicate a specific need for physical therapy. However, a patient with Down's syndrome may be referred if he or she has some type of orthopedic problem unrelated to the diagnosis.

162. A. Inferior glide is the correct mobilization technique to perform to increase abduction of the glenohumeral joint.

   Posterior glide would increase flexion and anterior glide would increase extension.

163. A. Limb synergies are necessary to the intermediate stage of recovery and should be encouraged to assist the patient. Brunnstrom's suggestion for therapy emphasizes eliciting motor behavior in the sequence in which it would normally occur following stroke, which is not the same as the sequence of normal maturation.

164. C. Cerebellar artery occlusion most likely results in coordination problems, as well as ataxia.

    A middle cerebral artery lesion would result in motor and sensory aphasia, as well as hemiplegia. A posterior cerebral artery lesion would result in loss of superficial touch and deep sensation, as well as contralateral hemiparesis. A vertebral artery lesion would result in loss of consciousness or coma.

165. C. Huntington's chorea is a hereditary condition characterized by chronic, progressive chorea and mental deterioration. No specific physical therapy treatment is required. In planning a treatment program for this patient, it would be appropriate to contact the family and suggest family education on the patient's conditions, as well as working with support personnel.

166. C. Scaphoid pads can be used to support the longitudinal arch and to assist in correction of pes planus.

    A Thomas heel is a heel with an extended anterior medial border used to support the longitudinal arch and correct for flexible pes valgus. Rocker bottom builds up the sole over the metatarsal heads and allows additional push-off in weak or inflexible feet. Metatarsal bars take pressure off the metatarsal heads by building up the sole proximal to the metatarsal heads.

167. B. Myositis ossificans is a rare, inherited disease in which muscle tissue is replaced by bone. It begins in childhood with stiffness in the neck and back and progresses to rigidity of the spine, trunk, and limbs. If the disease is active, then rest is the treatment of choice.

    However, if the disease is inactive, heat and gentle exercises may be prescribed.

168. D. Leg slides would be the least appropriate exercise to begin on day 1 post cesarean.

Diaphragmatic breathing, huffing, and pelvic floor exercises would all be appropriate to start on day 1.

169. C. Schizophrenia is a psychotic disorder in which the patient often has fragmented thoughts, bizarre ideas, and becomes withdrawn. Responses are usually inappropriate and demonstrate severe mood shifts.

Paranoia is a psychotic disorder in which the patient has delusions of persecution or grandiosity and is typically suspicious in all situations with all people. Depression is characterized by a feeling of sadness or helplessness. The patient typically has little drive for activity or achievement. Psychopathy is an antisocial personality disorder characterized by behavior patterns that lack moral and ethical standards.

170. C. The low-pressure mercury vapor lamp, otherwise known as cold mercury lamp, is utilized in application against the skin to kill bacteria.

The hot mercury lamp is a high-pressure mercury vapor lamp used for psoriasis skin conditions. It cannot be placed against the skin. The ultraviolet lamp is used in the control of infectious airborne bacteria and viruses, and in the treatment of psoriasis.

171. B. Capsular end-feel is characterized by hard leather-like stoppage with slight give. This will occur in full normal range of motion.

Bone-to-bone end-feel is defined by hard and abrupt stoppage to the joint motion. This typically occurs when performing passive range of motion and the bone contacts another bone. Empty end-feel is defined by a lack of stoppage to the joint. Springy block end-feel is defined by rebound movement felt at the end-range of passive range of motion. Two other end-feels include spasm end-feel and soft tissue approximation.

172. B. Flexor carpi ulnaris is innervated by the ulnar nerve.

Flexor pollicis longus, flexor digitorum superficialis, and flexor carpi radialis are innervated by the media nerve.

173. A. The dorsal scapular and long thoracic nerves originate from the rami of the plexus.

    The subclavian nerve originates from the trunk of the plexus. The lateral pectoral and musculocutaneous nerves originate from the lateral cord. The medial pectoral and ulnar nerves originate from the medial cord.

174. A. The best position for a joint in order to palpate the muscle would be a loose-packed position.

175. B. A left hemisphere cerebrovascular injury would result in paralysis and weakness on the left side.

    A cerebellar injury would result in ataxia, dysmetria, asthenia, and tremors. A brainstem injury would result in paralysis bilaterally and loss of consciousness.

176. C. Direct current is the only type of current that could be utilized to stimulate a denervated muscle. Direct current is necessary to get a response when stimulating a denervated muscle.

177. C. In performing goniometric measurement of the internal or external rotators of the shoulder, the stationary arm should be parallel or perpendicular to the midline of the floor. The moveable arm will then be longitudinally aligned with the shaft of the ulna and the styloid process. The axis for measurement is over the olecranon process.

178. A. One gram of fat yields 9 calories.

    One gram of protein yields 4 calories. One gram of carbohydrate yields 4 calories.

179. B. In order for distraction of the bodies to occur under lumbar traction, the therapist must apply traction from 40% to 50% of the body's weight.

180. D. Salicylate is an anti-inflammatory drug that utilizes the negative condition.

    Hydrocortisone, lidocaine, and magnesium are positive.

181. A. To perform an eccentric contraction, the muscle must lengthen as it develops tension. This is done through negative repetition. Another example would be lowering a weight during a hard press.

182. C. Under no circumstances is a physical therapist assistant able to provide initial evaluations on inpatients or outpatients.

183. A. Forced expiratory volume is air that can be forcibly expired after maximum inspiration.

    Forced inspiratory volume is the amount that can be forcibly inspired after maximum inspiration. Inspiratory capacity is the maximum volume inspired from the resting expiratory level. Tidal volume is the amount of air inspired and expired during a single breath.

184. D. Resting heart rate will decrease as a result of a cardiopulmonary training program that involves aerobic exercise.

185. A. Prolonged icing is utilized for the inhibition of muscles, while quick icing facilitates muscles.

186. C. Hypermobility is a precaution but not an absolute contraindication.

    Active inflammation, active infection, malignancy in the area of treatment, and recent fracture are absolute contraindications to mobilization. Precautions include joint effusion, rheumatoid arthritis, osteoarthritis, and presence of a bony block. Indications include joint dysfunction, restriction of movement, and pain.

187. D. In a prenatal care program the patient is encouraged to avoid Valsalva's maneuver. Valsalva's maneuver both increases pressure on the pelvic diaphragm and causes fluctuations in venous return to the heart.

    Kegel exercises are exercises for strengthening muscles of the pelvic floor. Activities of daily living modifications and relaxation training are all appropriate in a prenatal patient's program.

188. A. Crutch ambulation with toe touch weightbearing would be the most appropriate response for day 2 of a second-degree medial collateral ligament injury.

189. C. Partial curl-ups should not be performed secondary to not wanting to create a split of the rectus abdominis muscles that may develop before delivery.

    Diaphragmatic breathing, pelvic floor exercise, and postural instructions would be appropriate in a treatment program.

190. B. A patient with a lesion of T9 to T12 should have the functional outcomes of vital capacity 80%, be independent with floor to wheelchair transfers, perform gait with bilateral KAFO, and a walker.

    A patient with a lesion of T1 to T5 should have functional outcomes of vital capacity 80%, be independent in bed mobility without special equipment, and possibly be independent with bilateral KAFO and parallel bars. A patient with a lesion of L4-L5 should have functional outcomes of vital capacity 80%, be independent in bed mobility without special equipment, independent in transfers to and from the floor, and independent on all level surfaces. A patient with a lesion of T6-T8 should have functional outcomes of vital capacity 80%, be independent in bed mobility without special equipment, independent in a manual wheelchair on all level surfaces.

191. A. A first-class lever is best described when the fulcrum is located between the weight and the applied force. Examples in the body would be the atlanto-occipital joint or the action of the triceps at the olecranon.

    An example of a second-class lever is the pull of the brachioradialis muscle and wrist extensors on elbow flexion. With a third-class lever, the weight arm is longer than the force arm, designed for producing speed or for moving a small weight over a long distance. An example of a third-class level is the deltoid or glenohumeral joint. No fourth-class lever classification exists.

Definitions: Fulcrum: point of rotation
Force arm: distance of the lever between the joint (fulcrum) and muscle attachment—affect force
Weight: resistance arm—distance of the lever between fulcrum and weight

192. B. Intolerance to treatment as indicated by low $TcPCO_2$ values is an absolute contraindication to vibration of a neonate.

Persisted fetal circulation, increased irritability during treatment, and bradycardia are considered precautions.

193. C. Internal tibial torsion produces symptoms of the distal aspect of the tibia rotated or twisted medially as compared with its proximal end.

Anteversion results in the femoral neck rotated forward. Retroversion results in the femoral neck rotated posteriorly. In genu valgum, the tibia is angled laterally, causing the knees to come together.

194. B. The dermis layer is composed largely of a fibrous connective tissue that will bind the epidermis to the underlying tissues. Contained within the dermis are blood vessels and nerves.

The epidermis is the outer layer of the skin. It contains striated squamous epithelium cells. The epidermis functions to protect the underlying tissue against water loss, effects of harmful chemicals, and mechanical injury. The subcutaneous tissue is composed of adipose tissue.

195. B. For accurate crutch measurement, the patient should have approximately 20° to 30° of elbow flexion. This would be considered the one best answer. In a three-point gait pattern, weight is borne on the noninvolved leg, then on both crutches, then on the noninvolved leg. Touchdown and progression to full weightbearing on the involved leg are usual.

196. C. You should explain to the judge, or any patient, that as part of the physical therapist/client relationship, it would be unethical to accept a tip, although you appreciate his generosity.

197. D. Tinel's sign is an indication of irritability of a nerve, resulting in a distal tingling sensation on percussion of a damaged nerve. The sign is often present in carpal tunnel syndrome and is produced by tapping over the median nerve on the volar aspect of the wrist.

198. A. A Chi-square is a statistical test for an association between observed data and expected data represented by frequencies. The test yields a statement of the probability of the obtained distribution having occurred by chance alone.

Data is a collection of observations. Null hypothesis (HO) is a hypothesis that predicts that no difference or relationship exists among the variables studied that could not have occurred by chance alone.

199. C. Hip flexion is the least emphasized movement since most patients have adequate hip flexion and even have a tendency to develop contractures.

Chin tucks, pectoralis stretch, and shoulder flexion would all be areas of emphasis to maintain range of motion in a geriatric center.

200. B. When a patient is 7 to 9 months old, he or she should be able to sit alone, creep, or crawl and grasp with the thumb and forefinger.

When a patient is 10 to 12 months old, he or she should be able to cruise while holding onto furniture and stand and begin to walk. At 18 months, a child should be able to sit on a small chair.

Bibliography

Baxter R. *Pocket Guide to Musculoskeletal Assessment.* Philadelphia, Pa: WB Saunders; 1998.

Behrens BJ, Michlovitz SL. *Physical Agents in Theory and Practice for the Physical Therapy Assistant.* Philadelphia, Pa: FA Davis; 1996.

Bottomley J. *Quick Reference Dictionary for Physical Therapy.* Thorofare, NJ: SLACK Incorporated; 2000.

Curtis, K. *The Physical Therapist's Guide to Health Care.* Thorofare, NJ: SLACK Incorporated; 1999.

DeFranco J, Meyer T. *Outpatient Rehabilitation Certification Manual.* Hermann, Mo: Midwest Hi-Tech Publishers; 1998.

Fischback F. *Common Laboratory Diagnostics Test.* 2nd ed. Philadelphia, Pa: Lippincott; 1998.

Gogia P. *Clinical Wound Management.* Thorofare, NJ: SLACK Incorporated; 1995.

Goodman CC, Boissonnault WG. *Pathological Implications for the Physical Therapist.* Philadelphia, Pa: WB Saunders; 1998.

Guide to Physical Therapy Practice Act. Alexandria, Va: American Physical Therapy Association; 1999.

Hoppenfield S. *Physical Examination of the Spine and Extremities.* Norwalk, Conn: Appleton-Century Crofts; 1982.

Irwin S, Tecklin JS. *Cardiopulmonary Physical Therapy.* St. Louis, Mo: CV Mosby Co; 1995.

Kaufmann T. *Geriatric Rehabilitation Manual.* Philadelphia, Pa: Churchill Livingstone; 1999.

Kendall F, McCreary E. *Muscle Testing and Function.* 4th ed. Philadelphia, Pa: Lippincott, Williams & Wilkins; 1999.

Liebman M. *Neuroanatomy Made Easy and Understandable.* Gaithersburg, Md: Aspen; 1996.

Littell EH. *Basic Neuroscience for the Health Professions.* Thorofare, NJ: SLACK Incorporated; 1990.

Magee DJ. *Orthopedic Physical Assessment.* Philadelphia, Pa: WB Saunders Co; 1992.

Malone T, McPoil T, Nite A. *Orthopedic and Sports Physical Therapy.* 3rd ed. St. Louis, Mo: Mosby; 1997.

Merck Manual. Whitehouse Station, NJ: Merck Reseacrh Laboratories; 1996.

Michlovitz SL. *Thermal Agents in Rehabilitation.* 2nd ed. Philadelphia, Pa: FA Davis; 1990.

Molick, MH, Carr JA. *Manual on Management of Burn Patients.* Pittsburgh, Pa: Harmarville Rehab Center.

Monorkin CC, Levangie PK. *Joint Structure & Function: A Comprehensive Analysis.* Philadelphia, Pa: FA Davis Co; 1992.

Mosby's Medical Dictionary. 5th ed. St Louis, Mo: Mosby; 1998.

Normative Model of Physical Therapy Assistant Education Version 99. Alexandria, Va: American Physical Therapy Association; 1999.

O'Connor LJ, Gourley RJ. *Obstetric and Gynecologic Care.* 2nd ed. Thorofare, NJ: SLACK Incorporated; 1999.

O'Sullivan S, Schmitz T. *Physical Rehabilitation Assessment and Treatment.* Philadelphia, Pa: FA Davis Co; 1994.

Perry J. *Gait Analysis: Normal and Pathological Function.* Thorofare, NJ: SLACK Incorporated; 1992.

Rothstein J, Wolfs RS. *The Rehabilitation Specialist Handbook.* Philadelphia, Pa: FA Davis Co; 1998.

Scanlon V, Saunders T. *Essentials of Anatomy.* Philadelphia, Pa: FA Davis; 1994.

Scully R, Barnes M. *Physical Therapy.* Philadelphia, Pa: JB Lippincott Company; 1989.

Shannon M, Wilson BA, Stang CL. *Health Professionals Drug Guide 2000.* Stamford, Conn: Appleton and Lange; 2000.

Sullivan, Markos. *Clinical Decision Making in Therapeutic Exercise.* 1995.

Tabors Encyclopedia Medical Dictionary. 18th ed. Philadelphia, Pa: FA Davis; 1997.

Tecklin JS. *Pediatric Physical Therapy.* 3rd ed. Philadelphia. Pa: Lippincott; 1999.

Test Answer Form

EXAMPLES	IMPORTANT DIRECTIONS FOR MARKING ANSWERS
WRONG 1 ① ⊗ ③ ④ **WRONG** 2 ① ② ⊘ ④ **WRONG** 3 ① ② ③ ◑ **RIGHT** 4 ① ② ③ ●	• Use #2 pencil only. • Do NOT use ink or ballpoint pens. • Make heavy black marks that fill the circle completely. • Erase cleanly any answer you wish to change. • Make no stray marks on the answer sheet.

	A B C D		A B C D		A B C D		A B C D
1	① ② ③ ④	21	① ② ③ ④	41	① ② ③ ④	61	① ② ③ ④
2	① ② ③ ④	22	① ② ③ ④	42	① ② ③ ④	62	① ② ③ ④
3	① ② ③ ④	23	① ② ③ ④	43	① ② ③ ④	63	① ② ③ ④
4	① ② ③ ④	24	① ② ③ ④	44	① ② ③ ④	64	① ② ③ ④
5	① ② ③ ④	25	① ② ③ ④	45	① ② ③ ④	65	① ② ③ ④
6	① ② ③ ④	26	① ② ③ ④	46	① ② ③ ④	66	① ② ③ ④
7	① ② ③ ④	27	① ② ③ ④	47	① ② ③ ④	67	① ② ③ ④
8	① ② ③ ④	28	① ② ③ ④	48	① ② ③ ④	68	① ② ③ ④
9	① ② ③ ④	29	① ② ③ ④	49	① ② ③ ④	69	① ② ③ ④
10	① ② ③ ④	30	① ② ③ ④	50	① ② ③ ④	70	① ② ③ ④
11	① ② ③ ④	31	① ② ③ ④	51	① ② ③ ④	71	① ② ③ ④
12	① ② ③ ④	32	① ② ③ ④	52	① ② ③ ④	72	① ② ③ ④
13	① ② ③ ④	33	① ② ③ ④	53	① ② ③ ④	73	① ② ③ ④
14	① ② ③ ④	34	① ② ③ ④	54	① ② ③ ④	74	① ② ③ ④
15	① ② ③ ④	35	① ② ③ ④	55	① ② ③ ④	75	① ② ③ ④
16	① ② ③ ④	36	① ② ③ ④	56	① ② ③ ④	76	① ② ③ ④
17	① ② ③ ④	37	① ② ③ ④	57	① ② ③ ④	77	① ② ③ ④
18	① ② ③ ④	38	① ② ③ ④	58	① ② ③ ④	78	① ② ③ ④
19	① ② ③ ④	39	① ② ③ ④	59	① ② ③ ④	79	① ② ③ ④
20	① ② ③ ④	40	① ② ③ ④	60	① ② ③ ④	80	① ② ③ ④

	A B C D		A B C D		A B C D		A B C D
81	① ② ③ ④	101	① ② ③ ④	121	① ② ③ ④	141	① ② ③ ④
82	① ② ③ ④	102	① ② ③ ④	122	① ② ③ ④	142	① ② ③ ④
83	① ② ③ ④	103	① ② ③ ④	123	① ② ③ ④	143	① ② ③ ④
84	① ② ③ ④	104	① ② ③ ④	124	① ② ③ ④	144	① ② ③ ④
85	① ② ③ ④	105	① ② ③ ④	125	① ② ③ ④	145	① ② ③ ④
86	① ② ③ ④	106	① ② ③ ④	126	① ② ③ ④	146	① ② ③ ④
87	① ② ③ ④	107	① ② ③ ④	127	① ② ③ ④	147	① ② ③ ④
88	① ② ③ ④	108	① ② ③ ④	128	① ② ③ ④	148	① ② ③ ④
89	① ② ③ ④	109	① ② ③ ④	129	① ② ③ ④	149	① ② ③ ④
90	① ② ③ ④	110	① ② ③ ④	130	① ② ③ ④	150	① ② ③ ④
91	① ② ③ ④	111	① ② ③ ④	131	① ② ③ ④	151	① ② ③ ④
92	① ② ③ ④	112	① ② ③ ④	132	① ② ③ ④	152	① ② ③ ④
93	① ② ③ ④	113	① ② ③ ④	133	① ② ③ ④	153	① ② ③ ④
94	① ② ③ ④	114	① ② ③ ④	134	① ② ③ ④	154	① ② ③ ④
95	① ② ③ ④	115	① ② ③ ④	135	① ② ③ ④	155	① ② ③ ④
96	① ② ③ ④	116	① ② ③ ④	136	① ② ③ ④	156	① ② ③ ④
97	① ② ③ ④	117	① ② ③ ④	137	① ② ③ ④	157	① ② ③ ④
98	① ② ③ ④	118	① ② ③ ④	138	① ② ③ ④	158	① ② ③ ④
99	① ② ③ ④	119	① ② ③ ④	139	① ② ③ ④	159	① ② ③ ④
100	① ② ③ ④	120	① ② ③ ④	140	① ② ③ ④	160	① ② ③ ④

	A	B	C	D			A	B	C	D
161	①	②	③	④	181	①	②	③	④
162	①	②	③	④	182	①	②	③	④
163	①	②	③	④	183	①	②	③	④
164	①	②	③	④	184	①	②	③	④
165	①	②	③	④	185	①	②	③	④
166	①	②	③	④	186	①	②	③	④
167	①	②	③	④	187	①	②	③	④
168	①	②	③	④	188	①	②	③	④
169	①	②	③	④	189	①	②	③	④
170	①	②	③	④	190	①	②	③	④
171	①	②	③	④	191	①	②	③	④
172	①	②	③	④	192	①	②	③	④
173	①	②	③	④	193	①	②	③	④
174	①	②	③	④	194	①	②	③	④
175	①	②	③	④	195	①	②	③	④
176	①	②	③	④	196	①	②	③	④
177	①	②	③	④	197	①	②	③	④
178	①	②	③	④	198	①	②	③	④
179	①	②	③	④	199	①	②	③	④
180	①	②	③	④	200	①	②	③	④

NOTES

NOTES

NOTES

NOTES

NOTES

NOTES

NOTES

NOTES

NOTES

NOTES

NOTES

BUILD *Your Library*

This book and many others on numerous different topics are available from SLACK Incorporated. For further information or a copy of our latest catalog, contact us at:

**Professional Book Division
SLACK Incorporated
6900 Grove Road
Thorofare, NJ 08086 USA
Telephone: 1-856-848-1000
1-800-257-8290
Fax: 1-856-853-5991
E-mail: orders@slackinc.com
www.slackbooks.com**

We accept most major credit cards and checks or money orders in US dollars drawn on a US bank. Most orders are shipped within 72 hours.

Contact us for information on recent releases, forthcoming titles, and bestsellers. If you have a comment about this title or see a need for a new book, direct your correspondence to the Editorial Director at the above address.

Thank you for your interest and we hope you found this work beneficial.